The Emotional Labour of Nursing Rev

For Agnes and Frank Smith

Also by Pam Smith

THE EMOTIONAL LABOUR OF NURSING: How Nurses Care

SHAPING THE FACTS: Evidence-Based Nursing and Health Care (*co-edited with Trudi James, Maria Lorentzon, Rosemary Pope*)

The Emotional Labour of Nursing Revisited

Can Nurses Still Care?

2nd Edition

Pam Smith

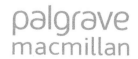

First edition 1992
Reprinted ten times
Second edition 2012

Palgrave Macmillan in the UK is an imprint of Macmillan Publishers Limited,
registered in England, company number 785998, of Houndmills, Basingstoke,
Hampshire RG21 6XS.

Palgrave Macmillan in the US is a division of St Martin's Press LLC,
175 Fifth Avenue, New York, NY 10010.

Palgrave Macmillan is the global academic imprint of the above companies
and has companies and representatives throughout the world.

Palgrave® and Macmillan® are registered trademarks in the United States,
the United Kingdom, Europe and other countries.

ISBN: 978–0–230–20262–7

This book is printed on paper suitable for recycling and made from fully
managed and sustained forest sources. Logging, pulping and manufacturing
processes are expected to conform to the environmental regulations of the
country of origin.

A catalogue record for this book is available from the British Library.

A catalog record for this book is available from the Library of Congress.

10 9 8 7 6 5 4 3 2 1
21 20 19 18 17 16 15 14 13 12

Printed and bound in Great Britain by the MPG Books Group,
Bodmin and King's Lynn

Contents

Illustrations

Acknowledgements

Throughout the second edition I have drawn on a number of research studies, and I would like to thank my co-researchers Helen Allan, Mike O'Driscoll, Maria Lorentzon, Ben Gray, Maureen Mackintosh, John Larsen and Leroi Henry. A number of publications have been forthcoming, and a complete list is available at the end of the reference list.

The original illustrations were compiled from a number of sources and feature in this second book. Thank you to the Department of Health, Cancer Relief Macmillan Fund (now Macmillan Cancer Support) and Marie Curie Cancer Care for permission to use their advertisements. The 'cartoon' was originally drawn by Cath Jackson as part of a series for Jane Salvage's book *The Politics of Nursing*. Thank you to both for permission to reproduce them here. A number of individuals contributed time and expertise to produce the photographs. They include Chris Priest of Magpie Reprographics and Liz Ashton Hill who took the photographs, the senior nurses who advised on locations and sources and the subjects who agreed to be featured. Recent photographs for 2011 were compiled from Thinkstock and iStock Photo collections.

In the 1992 edition, thanks go to the former English National Board of Nursing, Midwifery and Health Visiting (now the Nursing and Midwifery Council), for permission to reproduce extracts from the General Nursing Council's 1977 training syllabus and student nurse assessment form. I would also like to thank Dr Joan Fretwell for permission to use and reproduce her Ward Learning Environment Rating Questionnaire, Professor Martin Bland for his statistical advice and Professor Sally Redfern who supervised the original doctoral thesis on which the 1992 edition was based. Mike O'Driscoll adapted the questionnaire for the 2000s as an on-line survey.

I am grateful to Sheila Fawell for permission to include in the first book an extract from her study of student nurses undertaking their psychiatric experience. The findings of this study remain pertinent today.

Finally, I would like to thank Palgrave Macmillan and especially Lynda Thompson, Kate Llewellyn and Katie Rauwerda for their patience and belief in the need for a second edition of *The Emotional Labour of Nursing*. Thanks also go to Moyra Forrest for preparing the index.

Every effort has been made to trace all the copyright holders, but if any have been inadvertently overlooked, the publisher will be pleased to make the necessary arrangements at the first opportunity.

Preface

When I was invited by Lynda Thompson of Palgrave Macmillan to think about how to write a book about the 'Emotional Labour of Nursing' for the 2000s, after many hours of discussion we eventually agreed that the original book should remain 'intact' as a 'classic' text.

I clearly remember the incident that triggered me to make an in-depth study of nursing, which formed the basis of the book in the 1980s. I was working as a nurse teacher in an elderly care ward when a student told me that she had been reprimanded by the ward sister[1] for stepping out of the ward routine. The student had been so excited at being encouraged in the classroom to give patients choice that the sister's displeasure at having her ward routines disrupted came as quite of a shock.

The incident provoked a number of questions. What was it that compelled the sister to insist that certain tasks were completed by a regular time? Was it unreasonable to put patients at the centre of care? Most importantly, I felt I had let the student down. Was I promoting nursing ideologies that were inappropriate to the students' everyday realities? Somehow I didn't think so. But I had to find out why and how.

Eventually I was given the opportunity to seek answers by a progressive nurse manager who saw the value of an in-depth study of the subjective experiences of student nurses during training. As a participant observer I had a unique opportunity to talk to nurses and to be allowed back into the world of the ward. I experienced first hand some of the contrasts and contradictions of learning to care and was led to feel it, along with the nurses, as labour of an emotional kind.

Discussions after a sociology seminar with friends brought Arlie Hochschild's study of flight attendants to my attention. I would like to thank Anne Karp who told me about that study, *The Managed Heart*, which introduced me to the notion of 'emotional labour' as part of work. Her sociological imagination facilitated me not only in the writing of the book but also to extending my understanding of the notion of emotional labour as applied to nursing.

Finally, thanks to the student nurses, sisters, teachers and staff nurses in the first study for showing me what it means to care. Since then the changes within the health service towards a target-driven market, the move of nurse education into higher education and the impact of caring for people with long-term conditions have increased the emotional load on nurses. Their caring capacity is stretched to the limit. But the message remains the same: caring is work and requires skill and resources.

The opportunity to write a second book has allowed me to revisit the original emotional labour study and integrate commentaries on the basis of new research and policy analysis. This is the result. In the eight chapters that follow, I comment on the original case study material, re-examine some of the questions which asked 'how do student nurses learn to care' and re-consider emotional labour as a device for understanding how they learn and work. I present new research to ask 'can nurses still care?' The findings from the first study were used to construct a series of close-up portraits, nurses' own accounts and reflections on the nature of nursing and caring. Each chapter examined the viability of emotional labour as a concept, nurses' different emotional styles, the students' training trajectories and how they learnt to care, the role of the ward sister in setting the emotional tone, the legitimization of emotional labour and the forms it took between both nurses and nurses on the one hand and nurses and patients on the other and the strategies nurses adopted both to keep in touch and to protect themselves from their feelings.

New theoretical perspectives and empirical data are drawn upon in this second book to interrogate the original data and offer new insights into student nurses' experiences of learning nursing and caring in the dramatically changed educational and service contexts of the 2000s. Eight new chapters have been written which contain the original material, much of it intact but with substantial commentaries and analyses of student nurses' experiences of learning and caring in the contemporary health service.

Throughout the book I draw on studies I have been involved with over the past decade. Co-researchers helen allan, Mike O'Driscoll and Maria Lorentzon of the Centre for Research in Nursing and Midwifery Education, The University of Surrey and Ben Gray, former research fellow in the Faculty of Health, London South Bank University were involved in re-visiting and re-examining the emotional labour of nursing and how student nurses learn to care. John Larsen, former research fellow, the Centre for Research in Nursing and Midwifery Education, The University of Surrey, Leroi Henry, former research fellow, and Maureen Mackintosh, Professor of Economics, the Open University were involved in researching overseas nurses' experience of migration and governance and incentives in primary care, which opened up new areas of emotional labour research.

In 1992 I thanked many people for their inspiration and support. David Wield, Joe Hanlon, Teresa Smart and Maureen Mackintosh have continued to play a vital role in encouraging me to talk about and research emotional labour and ultimately to write this second book.

Since I wrote my original book, Arlie Hochschild has unstintingly provided the inspiration for further researching and understanding the complexities of emotional labour, its relationship to care and a re-conceptualisation for the global age. Arlie's generosity of time, presence and conversations have not only enriched me personally but also inspired the creation in 2000 of an emotional labour network with Steve Smith and Mike Rustin, Del Lowenthal, Ruth Simpson and Debbie Mazhindu. This network reaches to colleagues throughout the UK, Japan and the USA.

In drawing the second book to a conclusion, a number of key events have created an important backdrop. In July 2010, the Nursing and Midwifery Council consulted with the nursing profession on current educational provision in order to inform the revision of the educational curriculum in readiness for the new graduate level programmes required for 2013.

Furthermore, the political landscape is rapidly changing in response to the coalition government's 2011 plans to radically cut back public sector investment which many fear will transform the National Health Service away from its central values of a public service free at the point of delivery for all. Traditionally nursing has fared badly during economic downturns, revealing the susceptibility of the female workforce to market forces. This may well explain why nurses and nursing become scapegoats for the reported loss of compassion, empathy and caring relationships at the frontline of care.

This second book seeks to understand the contemporary context of nurses and nursing as portrayed through popular and professional rhetoric to re-examine the notion of emotional labour as a component of caring and learning to care. New evidence shows that nurses can still care, but that effort, skill and organizational support are required to ensure they can make a positive difference to carers and the cared for through those 'little things' that count for so much. This book is dedicated to them.

I was delighted that both Arlie Hochschild and Alan Pearson agreed to write forewords to the second edition of the Emotional Labour of Nursing. Arlie provides the sociologist's imagination and insight which comes from her original conceptualization of emotional labour and its costs. Alan as a leading nurse and academic in the UK and Australia is one of the key inspirations for person-centred care and evidence-based practice. Both Arlie and Alan are uniquely placed to provide a contemporary lens through which to view the emotional labour of nursing.

www.palgrave.com/nursinghealth/smith
- features the methodological appendices to the author's original and new research

Foreword

'Making little things big'

Making sure a hearing aid works. Eye glasses are clean. Fingernails clipped. Pam Smith refers to these as 'the little things' that matter to a patient. And to this list she might add a joke about hearing what we want to, a chat during the fingernail clip, a feeling of caring and being cared for. For Smith, empathy and attentiveness lie at the very core of nursing, and the systems should design themselves around that core.

This message was important when Smith's book first appeared in 1992, and is even more so now, not only in England where she conducted the highly moving interviews recorded here, but throughout much of Europe and the U.S. For today, we hear an ever louder call to cut government services, relax market regulation and transfer care facilities from public to for-profit hands.

This has not been good news for care. Indeed, under the high-flying banner of efficiency, many hospitals have squeezed out care. The Beth Israel Hospital in Boston, Massachusetts, U.S.A. , for example, was once a national beacon for professional 'total patient care'. Even mundane tasks were understood as part of a nurse's wider role which included evaluating, planning for, coordinating, and – in a full sense, giving – medical care.

But following a merger with another hospital, and restructuring, the hospital laid off many workers. Nurses were no longer assigned to given patients but instead floated from unit to unit depending on the number of filled beds. Physical tasks such as drawing blood, easing a post-operative patient onto a chair, escorting a crippled patient to the bathroom were redefined as 'menial' and assigned to unskilled and poorly paid workers. Turnover was high, and patients themselves had shorter stays. Acts of care did not find their way onto the patient's medical chart. And as someone remarked, 'If it isn't on the chart, it didn't happen.' The emotional labour of the nurse became invisible and its value quietly declined. Many nurses found themselves trying to protect their patients and themselves from life in a broken care system – itself a secondary form of emotional labour.[1]

The book in your hands holds out a radically more humane vision of care for the ill and frail. At its deepest level, Smith persuasively argues that, to care is a matter of heart-and-head-and-hand and of relating to the patient 'as a whole person'. The caring nurse is not caught in a speed-up. She's not glued to the computer monitor without time to look at the patient. She sees her relationship with the patient not as an impediment to healing but as a powerful part of it. She *feels good* about what she does and about the culture of care in which she works.

At its most profound level, this book is a call to the better angels of modern society. It is a call for raising high the standards of care, helping nurses to achieve it, and for healing the very system in which healing takes place. It's a book about making the little things big.

Arlie Hochschild
University of California, Berkeley

*   *   *

'Recognizing and valuing care'

Bev Taylor, an Australian professor of nursing in her study of 'ordinariness' in nursing, describes nursing as a human relationship that involves,

> ... all of the usual complexities of interhuman relationships, intensified even more by the extra effects of illness and the need for nursing care. Nurses are in unique positions, as people who have special knowledge and skills about people and their response to illness, and because they have front row seats to watch the dance of humanity; and, as such, they have the potential to make sense of human existence through close interactions with humans in need of care. (Taylor, 1994)

Another Australian professor of nursing, Ken Walsh, describes the importance of this relationship, referring to it as 'shared humanity'. In my very long career as a nurse, the elegance of nursing practice that encompasses this ability to engage with people in the caring process (be it, Taylor's words, joining in the dance of humanity or, Walsh's, engaging in shared humanity) has always intrigued me. Nursing others is indeed complex and draws on a range of sophisticated (and difficult to identify and describe) skills and actions that I have struggled to understand. My interest in this core of nursing has been central to all of the work I have pursued since entering nursing in 1964. There is, it seems to me, something about the therapeutic nature and power of the caring act of nursing another that has eluded us in our quest for understanding nursing itself and its role in health and healing.

Pam Smith's (1988; 1992) work on nursing as emotional labour played a significant role in my thinking about this centrality of the nurse–patient relationship in the delivery of healthcare and in drawing my attention to the emotional content of nursing in contemporary, high tech healthcare, and to the burden of labouring emotionally in an era where emotional labour is rendered invisible by our focus on effectiveness, efficiency, on outcomes and economics.

In her earlier work, Pam Smith drew on studies of flight attendants and debt collectors. In examining the core nature of nursing, she revealed to me that, although engagement in the practicalities of physical caring and curing is a critical component of nursing, the 'labour' of nurses is intrinsically emotional and requires the nurse to participate emotionally with those she or he cares for. My frustration with the over-emphasis on performing tasks and applying medical and bioscientific knowledge, and with the decentralization of the 'caring' part of nursing by policy makers, managers and nurses was – and still is – in part, explained. I learned that emotional work/labour is as crucial a component of nursing as the intellectual and physical.

This new book – which builds on Pam Smith's earlier work – moves it into this second decade of the twenty-first century, some twenty-plus years later. It examines contemporary nursing to re-examine emotional labour as a component of the nursing role by examining the literature and a plethora of research studies that have grown out of her earlier work. The differences between the rhetoric surrounding nursing and caring in the 1980s with contemporary times are surprising; but no less surprising is how little has truly changed in the recognition of the importance of the emotional labour of nursing (or its costs). In revisiting the original data and the notion of emotional labour presented in her first book, Pam Smith concludes that '... nurses can still care but that it requires effort, skill and organisational support ...' and that '... care has become a contested concept because of policy and organisational changes that have hierarchically spilt nursing between qualified nurses and health care assistants or aides. Nurses and nursing therefore need more than ever the support and commitment of leaders who set an emotionally caring tone and promote an organisational and educational system sensitive to the complex and financially driven world of the twenty-first century.'

I commend this insightful work and recommend it to anyone who has an interest in ensuring that the therapeutic nature and power of the caring act of nursing another is recognized as the intelligent and sophisticated core of effective health care, and that the emotional labour of such caring is recognized and valued.

Smith, P. (1988) 'The emotional labour of nursing', *Nursing Times*, 84, 44, 50–51.
Smith, P.(1992) *The Emotional Labour of Nursing: How Nurses Care*, Basingstoke: Palgrave Macmillan.
Taylor, B. (1994) *Being Human: Ordinariness in Nursing*, Melbourne: Churchill Livingstone.
Walsh, K. (1996) Being a Psychiatric Nurse. Unpublished PhD Thesis, Department of Clinical Nursing, University of Adelaide, Adelaide.

Alan Pearson A. M.
Professor of Evidence Based Healthcare and Executive Director,
The Joanna Briggs Institute, Faculty of Health Sciences,
The University of Adelaide, Australia.

Introduction

'The little things'

In the introduction to my first book I described my experience of making beds with a student nurse soon after she was allocated to an elderly care hospital, and my memory of her being close to tears because she felt that the old people were being treated like sacks of potatoes – hauled out and in of bed at the beginning and end of their day with no control over their destiny. This was a defining moment in my search to understand how student nurses learned to care (Smith 1992). Other students talked more positively about their experiences of elderly care, discovering that it was 'the little things' that made the qualitative difference to patients' lives – little things such as dressing in their own clothes, manicuring their nails, making sure their hearing aids worked and their glasses were clean. As one student put it, in the elderly ward, the functioning hearing aid was just as much a lifeline as the intravenous infusion to the postoperative patient on the acute surgical ward. On the elderly ward, the high-tech heroics were set aside and the little things became all important.

Over two decades later these elderly care wards have mostly disappeared and given way to residential nursing and care homes located primarily in the independent sector, as part of a general shift towards the commercialization of elderly care brought about by the 1990 NHS reforms. Student nurses in the 2010s now experience caring for elderly people in these settings both as part of their placements but also as off duty contract workers as a way to supplement their bursaries. Although the context has changed there is evidence to suggest that 'the little things' still matter.

From my own experiences as a young patient and as a student nurse I recalled that in acute wards, it was 'the little things' that made the qualitative difference, especially as to how I felt: the nursing assistant who, when I was a patient, broke hospital rules to bring me an Easter egg; the sister in the outpatient department who noticed me shivering in a wheelchair and tucked me up in a blanket; and my own nurse teacher who visited students on the wards and encouraged us to talk about our patients as individuals rather than cases. I reflected that all these people had shown personal interest in me and made me feel safe and cared for in an environment that was otherwise threatening, rigid and hierarchical.

Twenty years later my experience of care was not as a patient but as a carer of two increasingly ailing and elderly parents for whom 'the little things' continued to make a difference as to how they felt. They told me how important it was that professionals treated them as equals with life histories that mattered. Other examples were not unlike my own memories, involving care and attention of physical needs, which in turn impacted emotional wellbeing. During a visit to my mother in a rehabilitation unit, she described how the night before she had felt very cold. One of the nurses had noticed and promptly wrapped a blanket around her and brought her a hot cup of tea. The little things were also dependent on the ability of the staff to step outside routines, as the following incident illustrates. During a period of hot sunny weather, I arrived at the unit to find my mother along with other residents sitting in their wheelchairs under the trees with the staff, chatting companionably and sipping fruit juice in the natural surroundings of the gardens, free from institutional constraints.

In a follow-up study to explore emotional labour and student nurse learning in the 2000s (Allan et al. 2008a)[1] a third year student described noticing 'the little things' as a quality that not every nurse developed. She said: 'you notice the little things and not everybody does'. Recalling an incident from her current ward experience she gave the following example:

> One of the patients had his wedding anniversary yesterday, after being married 42 years. When his wife came in I wished her 'happy anniversary'. She was pleased I remembered and she said it made a difference.

Another student described that making a difference to patients meant:

> A lot of the little things and I quite like, definitely like chatting to patients and asking them if they're alright, if they slept okay, have they got any worries?

Noticing the little things was also described by a practice educator[2] as part of being a good mentor[3] and necessary for developing positive relationships with students. She said:

> I think the students value just being made welcome and little things like being shown where the off duty is and where they can put their coat and it's the buddy side of it, yeah. They do appreciate that.

But these 'little things', or 'gestures of caring', are still difficult to capture and they slip by unnoticed in the daily routines and the hustle and bustle of institutional life. When a patient is there 'for life' then the absence of these 'little things' is stark evidence of the lack of care.[4] The recognition of the 'little things' becomes more urgent as increasing numbers of older people are likely to spend their final years in institutions. For students the importance of the little things as evidence of good personal relationships both between themselves and their patients and in turn between their mentors and themselves has taken on a particular significance in the acute care setting, where patient throughput is high, and the combination of their supernumerary status and staff shift patterns may have lowered their integration within the ward team and feelings of continuity compared with the student apprentices in the first study, who constituted two-thirds of the workforce.

So why then when these things make such a difference to how people feel do we still refer to them as 'little'? One explanation lies in the continued stereotyping of care as women's 'natural' work, which keeps it invisible and undervalued and on the margins of high-tech medically defined work[5] – the background context in which the caring and learning takes place.

The reproduction of gender stereotypes was no better demonstrated in the 1980s than in the public images and perceptions of nurses and nursing. Attitude surveys reveal, for example, that the public identify 'alertness to the needs of others' as the mark of both the good woman and the good nurse (Oakley 1984). These attitudes reflect the patriarchal nature of nursing's origins, enshrined in the powerful image of Florence Nightingale.[6] Nightingale continues to capture the imagination, as a recent biography, *Florence Nightingale: The Woman and Her Legend* (Bostridge 2008), testifies. Over the intervening decades Mary Seacole, a Jamaican-Scottish healer, herbalist and business woman, once shunned by Nightingale and the Victorian establishment has risen to prominence to take her rightful place in nursing history. When the first book was written her story was little known and in many ways epitomized the marginalization and devaluation that black nurses subsequently experienced (Alexander and Dewjee 1984, Smith 1987, Baxter 1988, Smith and Mackintosh 2007). Seacole, who was well established in Jamaica, regarded it her duty as a loyal citizen of the Empire to travel to London to offer her services as a nurse in the Crimea. Although her offer was rejected, she used her own means to travel to the war zone and care for injured and dying soldiers. She returned to the UK almost penniless, but a group of grateful soldiers organized a concert to raise funds for her. There are now portraits of Seacole in the National Portrait Gallery and the Royal College of Nursing in London which testify to the work undertaken by the Jamaican Nurses Association and the annual Black History month. Over the past thirty years this has highlighted the achievements of Seacole and other prominent members of the black community to reveal their hidden history.

In the early 1990s, when I wrote my first book, nurse recruitment posters conveyed the predominant image of nurses, usually white women, as carers rather than technicians, special people who make a difference. 'Patients remember nurses' one poster states; another shows a little girl in a nurse's uniform holding

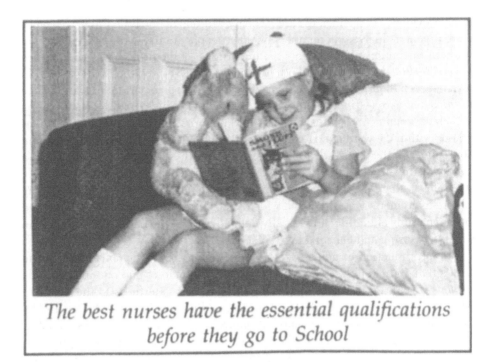

*The best nurses have the essential qualifications
before they go to School*

Illustration 1.1   Little girl in nurse's uniform with teddy bear
Note: This illustration is based on a DHSS recruitment advert from the early 1980s.
Source: Pam Smith.

her bandaged teddy bear: 'the best nurses have the essential qualifications before they go to school'. In other words, caring is portrayed as intuitive, instinctive, as something you're born with by virtue of your gender.

Young white women were still most likely to appear in the recruitment posters, and although a variety of technical images were presented (such as nursing a patient in head traction or tapping into a computer), the central message was that nursing is about people and ensuring the welfare of patients and their families.

By the mid-1990s, Kitson (1996), who at the time was a prominent nurse educator and researcher at the Royal College of Nursing, described the need for the images to change:

> The nurses of the future need new images to reconcile their technological skills with core values of caring and companionship.

A 1997 recruitment advertisement for general nursing had a 'Casualty'[7] like image of a pair of hands administering cardio-version therapy to the exposed chest of an unconscious patient. The caption read: 'Too much voltage and he dies, not enough and he dies. Clear?'

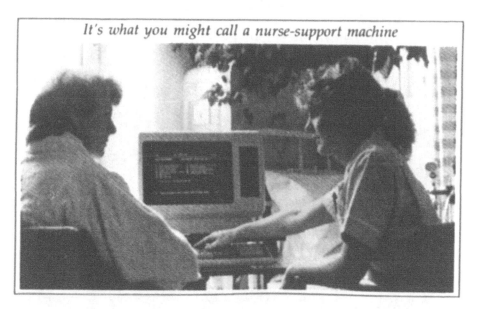

It's what you might call a nurse-support machine

Illustration 1.2   Nurse, patient and computer
Source: Department of Health. Reproduced with kind permission.

Technological skills were apparent in this message, in line with Kitson's recommendation, but not necessarily caring and companionship. Indeed the advert continued: 'You'll never forget the first time you bring someone back from the dead ... by punching a human heart back to life ... there's no other feeling like it'.

The requirements for such a job were specified as 'hard work, studying and decision-making'. In the corner of the picture, in small letters, the reader was asked 'Nursing. Have you got what it takes?' By focusing on the hands the advertisement was gender neutral, which suggested the importance of head and hand required in an emergency life-or-death situation, which took priority over the relational side to nursing, of care and companionship.

I detected another shift in the recruitment messages of the 2000s, which reflected nursing's move into higher education from the hospital schools of nursing where students are supernumerary rather than part of the workforce and supported by bursaries rather than wages. A recruitment poster from a London university, which asked 'At what price nursing?' assured prospective students that on completion of their three-year nursing programme they could expect the dual benefit of a good starting salary (£20,000 in 2005) and a university qualification.

This message is very much in contrast to the recruitment poster of the early 1990s, which gave a mixed message in response to the question 'Do the financial

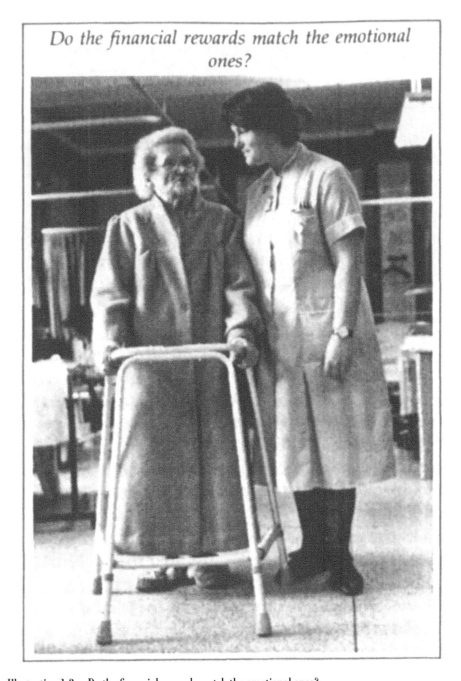

Illustration 1.3   Do the financial rewards match the emotional ones?

Note: This illustration is based on a DoH recruitment advertisement.

Source: Liz Ashton Hill. Reproduced with kind permission.

"MUMMY SAID SHE HAD CANCER. DADDY GOT VERY UPSET. THE NURSE MADE THEM BOTH FEEL BETTER."

A Macmillan Nurse helps care for people with cancer. We need your support to help her do even more. Send your donations to 15/19 Britten St, London SW3 3TZ.

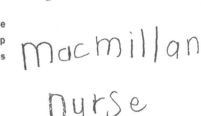

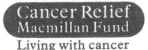

Cancer Relief
Macmillan Fund
Living with cancer

Illustration 1.4   Macmillan nurse with a smile

Source: Macmillan Cancer Support, formerly Cancer Relief Macmillan Fund. Reproduced with kind permission.

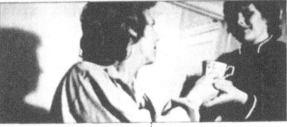

66It wasn't the cancer
patient who needed me it was the relatives.

When I arrived at the house the patient was asleep upstairs. I was immediately concerned about his wife. She looked as if she hadn't seen her bed for a week, which she probably hadn't.

Her daughter was just leaving as I arrived.

They were obviously very close, but I got the impression that the mother was still trying to protect the daughter, to shield her from what was happening. When we were alone, we talked. Just talked. About families, and how quickly things change. Sometimes a cup of tea is the best medicine in the world.

People sometimes ask me how I can do this, nursing people who are terminally ill. But you only have to take the hand of someone who's caring for a dying relative. Someone who's really desperate to rest. You can almost feel the relief easing its way through them. Then you know that it's worthwhile. 99

Every night Marie Curie nurses stay in the homes of people with cancer. They bring relief to the patients. And comfort and support to the relatives and friends who are caring for them. Please help us to continue this work.

I enclose a donation of £ _____ Please send me more
Information ☐ For credit card donations Tel: 071 823 1907

Name_____
Address_____

Postcode_____

To: Brian Roberts-Wray, Marie Curie
Cancer Care, 28 Belgrave Square,
London SW1X 8QG.

Illustration 1.5 Marie Curie nurse helps relatives

Source: Marie Curie Cancer Care. Reproduced with kind permission.

rewards match the emotional ones?' The answer (unlike the 2005 poster which directly addressed the issue of material reward) reassured prospective students on the one hand that although they were unlikely to be attracted to the job for the money, they could expect emotional rewards as well as financial ones. The conclusion here was that the emotional rewards came as an extra for working in one of the most 'emotionally satisfying careers'.

During the 1980s and early 1990s, when the first book was written, the cancer charities were prominent in promoting the nurse as a central feature of their services, with images of caring portrayed by holding, smiling nurses, who helped to ease the emotional pain of caring for a relative with cancer. One poster that advertised the nursing services of a cancer charity used a child's drawing of a smiling nurse with the caption: 'Mummy said she had cancer. Daddy got very upset. The nurse made them both feel better'.

An advertisement for the Marie Curie cancer charity showed three powerful images of a nurse comforting the distressed wife of a cancer patient. She was shown as performing the little things: holding, talking and preparing a cup of tea. The nurse seemingly performed these tasks effortlessly, with little demand on herself and for little material reward. Part of the wording read: 'People sometimes ask me how I can do this, nursing people who are terminally ill. But you have only to take the hand of someone who's caring for a dying relative. Someone who's really desperate to rest. You can almost feel the relief easing its way through them. Then you know it's worthwhile'.

These images suggest that when the first book was written the cancer charities were prominent in promoting the nurse as a central feature of their services with images of caring portrayed by holding, smiling nurses who helped to ease the emotional pain of caring for a relative with cancer. Over the past 20 years, this image has changed, as advances in cancer treatment has resulted in cancer being regarded, in many cases, as a long-term condition rather than a terminal illness. This is attributable, in no small measure, to the discoveries made about the role played by genetics, which makes it possible to find out whether a particular drug is likely to be effective based on the individual's genetic make-up. The advances in treatment and long-term management of cancer are reflected in the strategic vision and direction of the charities.

For example, the Cancer Relief Macmillan Fund, now renamed Macmillan Cancer Support, presents a broad strategic vision which includes proactive fund raising involving the public, fighting inequality and changing lives. Funding nurses is the first of seven strategic statements. Giving time, supporting families and making coffee can be identified as the indicators of emotional labour as a function of the whole organization. For example, a recent advertisement read 'Help with the Emotional Effects of Cancer' – 'We are Macmillan Cancer support', which suggested the organization had become the embodiment of that support through a corporate form of emotional labour.

Furthermore, since the first book was published, the IT revolution has had a massive impact on how information is transmitted to the public by means of websites and databases, and in the case of Macmillan Cancer Support a variety of booklets can be downloaded free from their website (www.macmillan.org.uk). In the context of emotional labour, two titles caught my eye; these were 'Hello and how are you?' and 'How are you feeling?' In addition public posters strategically placed at bus stops asked anonymous patients and their carers 'Are you tired of putting on a brave face?' Words rather than images were conveying the message, but in the booklets there were many powerful images of care and concern, laughter and determination, sincerity and concentration not only on the part of the professional but also on the part of the person with cancer and their carer. In some of the images it was not always possible to distinguish among professional, carer or person with cancer, which may be part of the power of the message being transmitted, that 'we are all in this together'.

Four areas were highlighted in the website of Marie Curie Cancer Care (www.mariecurie.org.uk): nursing, hospices, cancer research and palliative care research. Since the image in the first book was on the transmission of emotional labour by the nurse, I also focused on the section of the website demarcated as 'Marie Curie Nurses: How can we help?' The information given was that Marie Curie nurses and health care assistants (HCA)[8] care for 50 per cent of people with cancer who die at home and also for people with other end-of-life conditions 'every minute of every day'. Marie Curie Cancer Care continues to convey the message that their nurses support carers by allowing them 'to rest knowing that their loved-one is in safe hands' and support them 'at what can be an emotional and stressful time'. The accompanying booklet that can be downloaded carries images of concerned, considered and smiling patients, their carers and uniformed professionals. The emotional tone of the text both in the booklet and on the website was one of supportive partnership, while at the same time giving the sense of drawing a discrete boundary between the organization and the individual in contrast to the much more encompassing message of Macmillan Cancer Support, which conveys empowerment and partnership. It may even be possible to 'Be. Macmillan' and for professionals and public alike to create their own materials and resources.

What is care?

In the 1980s and 1990s I asked what is care? My second question in the context of these powerful images of nurses as caring (smiling, holding, talking) women, making things better for others was how can it be defined to go beyond such images? A number of feminist sociologists attempted to answer this question (Stacey 1981, Graham 1983, Ungerson 1983a, 1983b, 1990). Graham, for example, described caring as both labour and love, caring for and caring about, doing and feeling. She says: 'everyday conversations about caring are ... conversations about feelings. When we talk about caring for someone we are talking about our emotions' (Graham 1983, p. 15).

In general, caring relationships are those involving and defining women in both the public and private domain. Throughout the life-cycle women care for children, partners, relatives who are sick, handicapped or the elderly.[9] They reproduce these caring activities in the public arena of work.[10] But differences occur in the affective domain, where feelings of love, concern and empathy are in danger of being replaced by 'social distance' (Graham 1983).

Nicky James (1989), a nurse sociologist, who spent five months as a participant observer in a hospice, chooses to describe care as labour. She found that the demands of emotion work with the dying and their families could be as hard as physical and technical labour, but not so readily recognized and valued. James concludes that 'the management of emotions has many of the connotations associated with labour as productive work but also the sense of labour as difficult, requiring effort and sometimes pain. It demands that the labourer gives something of themselves and not just a formulaic response'.

She describes how emotions such as grief, anger, loss, despair and frustration were painful to watch and awkward to respond to, particularly as they did not fit in with standard ideas of workplace skills. But they were anticipated and seen as appropriate responses in coming to terms with death. Sometimes, however, nurses would choose to concentrate on the physical aspects of the patient's care in order to avoid difficult relationships. When this happened, the 'love' part of the work was lost (James 1986).

Arlie Hochschild (1983), an American sociologist, whose groundbreaking work was the inspiration for my doctoral research and first book, also makes conceptual links among care, feelings and emotions. In her study of flight attendants, Hochschild used the term 'labour' rather than 'care' to describe the emotional component of their work (smiling, friendly, kind, courteous) which was required as part of their job and had explicit monetary value both for themselves and the airline.

Hochschild defines emotional labour as 'the induction or suppression of feeling in order to sustain an outward appearance that produces in others a sense of being cared for in a convivial safe place' (p. 7). She goes on to say that jobs which involve emotional labour share three characteristics:

1. Face-to-face or voice contact with the public.
2. They require the worker to produce an emotional state in another, e.g. gratitude, fear.
3. They allow the employer through training and supervision to exercise a degree of control over the emotional activities of the employees (p. 147).

Thus, according to Hochschild, emotional labour is the occupational equivalent of emotion work/management which is done in a private context. It is sold for a wage and has exchange value. Because jobs with high components of emotional labour are most likely to be female occupations, gender stereotypes and expectations are reproduced in the workplace. Whether emotional labour is undertaken in the workplace or as emotion work/management in the home, it is guided by what Hochschild calls 'feeling rules'. Feeling rules are the scripts or moral stances that guide our action. They come from within us, the reaction of others and social conventions.

Emotion work/management/labour intervenes to shape our actions when there is a gap between what we actually feel and what we think we should feel. Take the feeling of 'anger', for example. 'Perhaps women are not any less aggressive than men', Flax, a feminist writer, suggests, 'we may just express our aggression in different, culturally sanctioned (and partially disguised or denied) ways' (1987). In order to express our feelings in 'culturally sanctioned ways', Hochschild suggests that there are two kinds of emotion work: surface and deep acting.

In surface acting, we consciously change our outer expression in order to make our inner feelings correspond to how we appear. Deep acting requires us to change our feelings from the inside, using a variety of methods such as imaging, verbal and physical prompting so that the feelings we want to feel show on our face. Both feeling rules and emotion work may be unconscious or semi-conscious. Subsequently, a number of scholars have put the emotional labour analysis of feeling rules, surface and deep acting within public and private care work under scrutiny. Hochschild also shifted her analysis to a focus on care, which she defined as 'an emotional bond' between carer and cared for as testified in the following citation:

> Most care requires work so personal, so involved with feeling that we rarely imagine it to be work. But it would be naive to assume that giving care is completely 'natural' or effortless. Care is the result of many small subtle acts, conscious or not (cited from Ruddick 1989).

Hochschild has since suggested that the commercialization of care work in a globalized economy has resulted in a 'care deficit' articulated through four distinct models which she suggests 'appear in public discourse on social policy and so provide a tool for decoding that discourse' (2003, p. 218).[11]

The emotional labour of care

But is emotional labour as a concept the same as care? What are the similarities and differences and the inherent contradictions of treating emotional labour as a commodity? In the first book I applied the concept of emotional labour to nursing because nurses are expected to be emotionally caring and display emotional styles similar to those of flight attendants.

I first experienced caring as labour during interviews with students and patients when the language that they used and the feelings that they expressed conveyed a sense of the sheer emotional work required to sustain the traditional image of smiling nurses, holding patients' hands. During one such interview a student described the following incident:

> I've had times when I've been with another nurse and we've been changing a patient's bed and he's shouted at her or been rude or something. Well the procedure goes on as if nothing has happened. And when we've finished she just drifts off. And I actually go after her and say 'Are you alright? I would have been very unhappy if he'd said that to me'. I think it's so important that we notice each other's distress so that we don't have to cry alone in a corner.

As this account demonstrates, nurses laboured emotionally not only for patients but also for each other. The ward sister was the key person who set the tone for the caring climate on her ward. As one student explained, 'if sister cares then I don't need to take the whole caring attitude of the whole ward on my shoulders'.

Bone (2009, p. 57), writing in the 2000s, talks about the changes in the US health care system where 'cost containment, medical control and profit making' have eclipsed 'those types of work that prioritize interpersonal and psychosocial care' and the negative effects these changes have had on nurses' emotional labour. Bone differentiates between 'instrumental' emotional labour characteristic of flight attendants' work and 'therapeutic' emotional labour, which is nurses' preferred style. Bone concludes that under harsh market conditions, nurses are forced to alter the style of care they give so that patients are left with no option other than to learn to live without it. She attributes this state of affairs to the conversion of many health and human services into commodities, which in turn reduce the availability of both paid and unpaid carers with the capacity to care, resulting in a 'care deficit'. In the context of the US, the results of harsh market conditions on health and human services are very obvious to Bone, but similar effects are becoming increasingly apparent in the UK and elsewhere.

Bolton's theoretical developments of emotional labour over the past decade (Bolton 2000, 2001, Bolton and Boyd 2003) have made useful contributions to unravelling the complexity of emotions in health care in general and nursing in particular. Bolton proposes a typology of workplace emotions and a range of motivational factors at individual and organizational level.[12] What particularly appealed to me in Bolton's analysis was the idea of emotional labour as a gift given for 'philanthropic' reasons by the gynaecology nurses, reminiscent of the 'gift relationship' described by Titmuss in his classic study of blood transfusion

(Titmuss 1970). The nurses described the use of humour in a therapeutic way, giving the patients the opportunity to have a laugh in an 'emotionful place' that was a 'woman's world', while a ward sister recognized the central role of curing to nursing when she said, 'The essential basis of nursing is caring. You can't be a nurse if you don't care' (Bolton 2000, p. 583).

Theodosius (2006, 2008) claims that emotion management, although conceptually innovative in its time, has potentially limited the relational aspects of emotion, in particular the unconscious processes taking place during patient-nurse interaction. She also reveals that working with emotions is integral to the way in which nurses construct their personal identity which goes beyond external factors to the very reasons why they choose to do nursing in the first place such as 'unconscious love' (Theodosius 2006, p. 899).

Theodosius (2006) decided therefore to apply a methodology that recovered the unconscious emotions by applying an interactive and unconscious approach in the field working with patients, nurses and other health care professionals to capture hidden and invisible emotion processes using diaries, interviews and participant observation. Theodosius was concerned that the emotional labour research undertaken by Nicky James and myself, rather than exposing emotion work and making it visible, had resulted in marginalizing it and driving it underground. Rather I would argue that the time when we were first researching and writing about emotions and nursing, we hit a spot that revealed a hidden world of nursing and learning to be a nurse. Subsequently, emotional labour as a concept has become 'normalized', and part of the everyday language of nursing and care work is being incorporated into the current discourse of compassion and dignity.

Theodosius (2008) has extended the analysis of emotional labour to examine the nature of emotions that nurses feel and how they form a part of their social identity, which goes beyond the presentational symbolic forms expressed through the emotion management framework first inspired by Hochschild (1983).[13] She demonstrates her approach through a series of powerful vignettes in which she sums up that 'therapeutic' emotional labour (which she distinguishes from 'instrumental' emotional labour) 'is still an important component to nursing care, that is still central to the nursing identity and that society in the form of those nurses care for – still needs and believes in it' (Theodosius 2008, p. 172). In these vignettes Theodosius deals with and describes complex and challenging situations where nurses are working at the extremes: from loving care to complaints; from trust and reciprocity with patients to feeling to be working at 'half measures' and being bullied by colleagues. This summary does not do justice to Theodosius' in-depth analysis, but she highlights the essential nature of two-way relationships between nurses, patients and their carers which contribute to the emotional labour process.

Scholars in a number of countries other than the UK have shown increasing interest in the application of emotional labour to nursing. Bone's (2009) study is just one of several examples from the USA. In Japan a translation of 'The Emotional Labour of Nursing' appeared in 2001, and interest continues to grow. The translator, Professor Asako Takei, has since published her own study of emotional labour (Takei 2001), and a number of collaborations and exchange visits with scholars and practitioners in Japan have ensued including symposiums and a public lecture attracting 300 delegates (Ars Vivendi 2009, Smith 2010, Smith and Cowie 2010). The appeal of emotional labour in the Japanese context is that it gives a language to describe feelings and behaviours that are recognized by practitioners, educators and researchers but are not always permitted by professional mores and circumscribed by public demands and expectations. The connections and differences between emotional labour and the more recent concept of emotional intelligence have also been explored.

Emotional labour and emotional intelligence

Emotional intelligence was first described at length by Goleman (1995). Huy (1999) makes theoretical connections between emotional labour and emotional intelligence and suggests that particularly at times of change, the process can be facilitated by judicious attention to emotions (Huy 1999). He concludes that emotions are an integral part of adaptation and change, and emotionally intelligent individuals are able to recognize and use their own and others' emotional states to solve problems. Huy identifies 'hope as an attribute of emotional intelligence and implies a belief that one has both the will and the means to accomplish one's goals. It buffers people against apathy and depression and strengthens their capacity to withstand defeat and persist in adversity'.

In the nursing literature, Freshwater and Stickley (2004) suggest that emotional intelligence and the capacity to care influence nursing behaviours and the delivery of care. Emotional intelligence is, they suggest, also linked to what students understand nursing to be and what student nurses learn to do as nurses. In relation to learning and socialization in nurse education, Akerjordet and Severinsson (2004) suggest that supervised learning in clinical practice for mental health students fosters emotional intelligence, responsibility, motivation and a deeper understanding of patient relationships and their identity and role as mental health nurses. Clouder (2005) has linked emotions and learning and suggests that concepts such as caring are particularly troublesome because the messiness of practice conflicts with the ideals students hold of caring; indeed they would like learning to care to be trouble free! But it is exactly this messiness where learning occurs and where emotions are a fruitful and creative part of learning (Allan et al. 2008b, pp. 550–1).

Nursing and care

But in what way do nursing leaders and educationalists conceptualize care, and do emotional labour and, more recently, emotional intelligence feature in this conceptualization? A look at the literature of the 1980s and 1990s showed an increasing emphasis on the emotional aspects of caring and its promotion as distinctly nursing work ever since the influential Briggs report of the early seventies (DHSS 1972).

Baroness Jean McFarlane, one of the UK's first prominent nursing academics, in a keynote address to the Royal College of Nursing, maintained that the words 'nursing' and 'caring' have similar roots. She says: 'Caring signifies a feeling of concern, of interest, of oversight, with a view to protection. Nursing means ... to nourish and cherish' (McFarlane 1976, p. 189).

McFarlane wanted to see an end to the nurse as the doctor's handmaiden and wanted to see the emergence of a new role in which caring was pre-eminent. By describing nursing in terms of 'helping, assisting, serving, caring for' patients, McFarlane was seeking to raise the status of so-called basic tasks to the level of unique nursing skills. In a subsequent paper, she provided a philosophy and work method called the nursing process, to do this (McFarlane 1977). The nursing process, regarded by many as an American import, promotes a people-orientated rather than a task-orientated approach to patients and raises the profile of emotional care at the same time that, as Hochschild notes, the growth of the service sector and 'people jobs' has made communication and encounter the central work relationship.[14]

Changes in the structure and knowledge base of nurse education proposed by the United Kingdom Central Council's Project 2000 (UKCC 1986) and innovations such as primary nursing described by Jane Salvage (1990) as part of the 'new nursing', built on the nursing process philosophy and work method to emphasize people-centred care rather than patients and disease.[15]

From the perspectives of the early 1980s, it appeared that the nursing leadership failed to grapple with the conceptual complexity of defining care, especially in relation to its emotional components and demands. An important implication of raising the profile of emotional care can be seen in the light of research undertaken in a London hospital over 50 years ago by Isabel Menzies, a British psychoanalyst, which has now finally been taken on board as a definitive piece of research in the nursing literature. Brought in to investigate some of the reasons why students were leaving nursing, she believed that high anxiety levels were partly responsible. Menzies saw the task-orientated way in which nursing care was organized as a defence against that anxiety (Menzies 1960). She wrote:

> The nursing service attempts to protect the nurse from the anxiety of her relation with the patient by splitting up her contacts with them. The total workload of a ward or

department is broken down into lists of tasks, each of which is allocated to a particular nurse.

In the light of Menzies' findings, the nursing process, with its explicit commitment to the development of nurse–patient relationships, could be seen to put nurses at risk of increasing their anxiety by removing the protection provided by task-orientated care.

The nursing leadership of the seventies and eighties also failed to address why many nurses favoured high-tech, medically defined nursing. McFarlane, for example, believed that an early job analysis of hospital nursing by Goddard (1953), in which the physical, technical and affective aspects of nursing had been distinguished, emphasized the status of technical over physical and affective nursing. Fretwell (1982) more realistically points out that the distinction reflected the existing medical division of labour and hierarchy within nursing. McFarlane's reaction was typical of the curious lack of feminist perspectives brought to bear on the position of nurses by its leaders. Issues such as the stereotyping of care as women's 'natural work' (encapsulated by the recruitment posters) and the gender division of labour within the health service and the patriarchal power relations between doctors (predominantly men) and nurses (predominantly women) were not addressed in these official versions of nursing.[16] *The Politics of Nursing*, written by Jane Salvage (1985), in which she addresses some of these fundamental issues, is an important departure from the traditional nursing texts.[17]

Nurse leaders who were firmly grounded in academic scholarship, politics and higher education were interviewed in the follow-up study in order to get a sense of where the leadership for learning was coming from (Allan et al. 2008a). They were clear that nursing had to keep pace with educational, organizational and global changes, which over the intervening decades had resulted in the need to look at nursing and nursing students from different perspectives. One leader took the view that student nurse learning and leadership was implicitly at the forefront of the new NHS because changing workforce initiatives since 1997 demanded new ways of working and shared learning among professions (Melia 2006). On the one hand policy reforms had led to 'the shaping of the nursing agenda by medical concerns, the main one being the desire for a (medical) consultant led service' and the establishment of a diversity of roles and nurse-led services on the other. These reforms have not necessarily been accompanied by structural, organizational and educational changes required to change professional cultures and patient empowerment to meet the challenges of the new workforce. The gap in being able to educate the next generation of practitioners in these new roles is borne out by a former ward sister reflecting on her transition to clinical nurse specialist (Mann 1998) in which she observed that the emphasis on student nurse learning in her new role had diminished.

Another leader suggested that students 'want to go as far as they can to work at the interface with medicine and push role boundary work to its limit' requiring both educators and students to 'think outside the box' in order to meet these different aspirations and to pioneer different approaches and models of practice. Thinking differently assisted students to craft and create their own learning environment 'wherever that happens to be'. The leader concluded that flexible and innovative approaches to learning and practice were necessary because the 'temporal order of the delivery of care has changed as have the spaces in which it is delivered'. Finally, she challenged the interviewer's assumption that the opportunities to think were constrained by the ward environment because, in her view, the role of the clinical leader was to encourage students to think dynamically in order to build their capacity to transcend boundaries, people and roles. She said:

> There are people that you find it easier to think with and places where thinking is more legitimately recognised. But I think if you are curious, you're just curious and you sort of express that regardless of where you happen to be, although it helps when the environment and the context and the culture are right for it.

The need to go beyond traditional boundaries and stereotypes to think outside the box was expressed by another leader who prioritized values-based nursing and 'altruistic behaviour' as 'going beyond the job descriptions':

> I like to think that you should or could have qualities that go beyond just the job descriptions to achieve a fully rounded set of skills to deal with people in a comprehensive way.

The importance of passing on knowledge and clinical skills was highlighted by a third leader committed to fostering an 'intergenerational approach' to encourage alumni to mentor future students in a variety of educational settings whether in the classroom, specially designed clinical skills laboratories or the clinical areas which put caring at the core. Such an approach required skill mix models that built in 'opportunities for qualified nurses to be deeply involved in care' as well as dealing with their management responsibilities to deal with budgets, targets and other bureaucratic requirements.

The body–mind dichotomy

Concepts of care continue to be fraught with contrasts and contradictions and generate a range of questions. Is it labour or is it love? Is it natural or is it a skill? Is it about feelings or tasks? Does it come from the heart, the head or the hand? Is it guided by mind or body? Or can caring be seen as an integrated whole? In response to this last question the nurse leaders whose views are reported above are clear that it should. One leader raised an additional question which arose from the 'check box' culture with its emphasis on clinical competences in which

> you get to the point that you only measure and have interest in the things you can tick, then what happens to qualities such as judgement and integrity? You can't tick either of those because they'd take time to mature and it's about how the practitioner *feels about* what they are doing and have the opportunity to reflect on their practice (my emphasis).

Because of the heightening awareness of the need for nurses to be able to be given emotional spaces to think and feel about their practice highlighted by these contemporary leaders, there have been some criticisms of Hochschild's work which described emotional labour as a 'technical fix' and perpetuating the body–mind dichotomy, with its origins in positivism, western dualism and what Mary O'Brien calls 'male-stream' thought.[18] Pat Benner, an American Professor of Nursing, applies a philosophical approach to the concept of care, which she says transcends the body–mind split and enables connection and concern between nurse and patient. Emotions are seen as the key to this connection because 'they allow the person to be engaged or involved in the situation .... The alienated, detached view of emotions, as unruly bodily responses that must be controlled actually cuts the person off from being involved in the situation in a complete way' (Benner and Wrubel 1989).

Views such as these represent a trend apparent in the 1980s among nurses in the USA and Europe to move to a more holistic approach to care and away from 'a nation's blind embrace of high tech medicine' (Gordon 1988).

This trend towards holistic care has continued over the intervening decades with increasing attention to the role of emotions in nursing and caring. Three characteristics of this trend can be noted. The first characteristic illustrated by Theodosius' work is the role of the unconscious and psychoanalytic and psychodynamic approaches to emotions. Phenomenology and embodiment as characterized by Benner's work continues to be acknowledged as important for nursing. The symbolic interactionist and Marxist stance of the cognitive approach to emotions characterized by Hochschild's work has attracted increasing theoretical critiques, in particular the risk that emotions become normalized and thus maginalized which detracts from what is given 'freely' as part of who one is and what one is paid to do (McClure and Murphy 2007).

My own empirical work refutes this view as one that can encourage nurses and women to give over and above what they are supported to do both personally and professionally. The emotional labour analysis pays attention to the division of labour within the health service and the gendered nature of care and has been expanded by Hochschild to examine the notion of a 'care deficit', which goes beyond the individual to systems and processes and the wider society in which nurses and others operate to reveal how care as a core value has become increasingly threatened and devalued.

The politics of care

As concerns for cost-effectiveness and efficiency sweep the British health service and budgets are finely tuned to respond to the purchaser–provider divide, the little things are in double danger. On the one hand, nurses working under increasing pressure will find even less time to do the little things for patients. On the other, the increase in monitoring and standard setting may focus more on quantitative measures rather than on qualities of care. At what price is care, since emotional care is not easily costed?

A 1990s recruitment poster gave a mixed message. On the one hand, it reassured prospective nurses that although they were unlikely to be attracted to the job for the money, they would be well paid for their skills. On the other hand, it emphasized that they could expect emotional rewards *as well as* financial ones. In other words, the emotional rewards came as an added bonus for working in one of the most emotionally satisfying professions (see illustration on p. 7).

It was interesting to speculate that at the time of writing the first book, there appeared to be a trend towards the privatization of the NHS and a fear that this would lead to the commercialization of nurses' emotional labour in the private health industry. There were images already being used for advertising private health insurance in the early 1990s, which bore similarities to those used by the airline industry to attract customers in the days before low-budget, 'no frills' airlines. Like the recruitment posters and charity advertisements of the 1990s, the nurse in the private sector was also portrayed as the key carer, smiling and helpful to the patient and their family (see illustrations on above pages and below).

At the same time, a contradictory trend was emerging in the rapidly changing health service of the 1990s which tended to marginalize care even further from medically defined work. An example is a *Guardian* article at the time, which described an elderly care ward staffed by untrained carers (Brindle 1990). Nurse training was criticized for being too formal and nurses too wedded to routine to provide the 'caring touch' for elderly long-stay residents. The technical needs of the residents were provided by a visiting nurse who was described as doing the 'tricky dressings' and complicated medicines. The untrained carers on the other hand described themselves as 'just making people happy' which in a health service sensitive to cost efficiency and effectiveness, drove a sharp division between caring and technical requirements, potentially marginalizing the little things or caring gestures, from technical skills. By the 2000s the division between caring and technical nursing had become even more sharply defined.

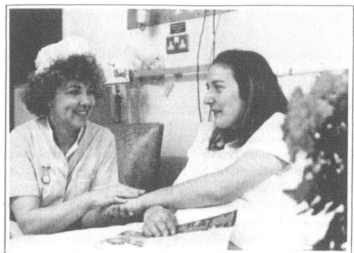

Feel confident that when you or a member of your family need
hospital treatment, you'll enjoy comfort, privacy and individual
attention.

**Illustration 1.6   A nurse in full dress uniform and frilly cap gives 'individual attention' to a patient
paying for private hospital care**

Note: This illustration is based on a private health insurance advert.

Source: Liz Ashton Hill. Reproduced with kind permission.

By 2008, the health care assistant (HCA) had become firmly established on
the lowest rung of the nursing hierarchy to deliver frontline care, drawing on
existing precedents for unqualified nursing labour (the untrained carer, the
nursing auxiliary or the student nurse) to support the work of registered nurses
(Dewar and Macleod-Clark 1992, Thornley 2001). Project 2000 demanded
the withdrawal of student nurses from the frontline workforce, where they had
formerly given up to 75 per cent of direct patient care (Moores and Moult
1979), to become supernumerary with perceived benefits to their learning
(UKCC 1985). The introduction of the NHS Plan (Department of Health
2000) lent further support to the establishment of HCAs as the main players
in the delivery of frontline care. The Plan proposed increasing their numbers,
expanding the role and allocating a dedicated training budget to facilitate
their progression via the National Vocational Qualification (NVQ) scheme
and initiatives to meet local workforce needs (Department of Health 2003a,
2003b). Even though the HCA might be trained to work at a relatively senior
level in a prestigious speciality such as critical care, Johnson et al. (2004)
found that the main aspiration of the role was still to 'relieve qualified nurses
from routine, if far from basic tasks and procedures'. According to one nurse

leader, organizing the division of labour in this way has created a dilemma for nursing because:

> Students are no longer the workforce providing basic care; HCAs are doing this and students no longer seek to do basic care; they seek to instruct others to do it rather than have a lifetime of doing it. The role of the staff nurse is the management of care, administration, organization and communication outside the ward.

For another nurse leader, taking staff nurses away from direct patient care placed them in a contradictory situation with regards to the education of student nurses and their effective supervision, in that leaders of nursing needed to give care in order to know how to supervise it.

Dividing labour in this way coincides with the introduction of targets within the NHS, which has changed and focused the organization of health care so that there is speed up and an emphasis on rapid throughput within the acute sector and the management of chronic illness and personal and social care within community and primary care (Ross et al. 2009).

As if to counteract targets and subsequent speed up, a recent trend within the health service is to promote dignity and compassion (Smith 2008). This trend has taken on different perspectives in England and Scotland. In England, a compassion index, the first of several initiatives proposed in the NHS Review *High Quality Care for All* (Department of Health 2008), scores how compassionate nurses are towards patients. Components of compassion include indicator smiles, and by inference the emotional labour defined by Hochschild (1983) as 'the induction or suppression of emotions to make others feel safe and cared for', which is required to give empathetic care (Smith 2008). The compassion index also includes measures of good nutrition, hand washing and safety as key indicators of quality care.

In Scotland, a project to enhance 'patient care by promoting compassionate nursing practice' was set up and supported by a local businesswoman, the local Health Board and a local university (www.napier.ac.uk/fhlss/NMSC/compassionatecare). One of the key strands was to support the development of leadership skills to provide compassionate care in a range of care settings. Meeting with the senior nurses involved in the project revealed a high level of commitment to and enthusiasm for identifying and describing compassionate care through narratives triggered by emotional touch points (Bate and Robert 2007, Dewar et al. 2010). Capturing stories showed the impact emotions had on patients, carers and professionals and the positive and negative effects that enhanced or hindered compassion. A textbook for carers, students and practitioners of nursing and health visiting described compassion as 'the key to rediscovering what lies at the heart of nursing practice' that would assist readers develop their 'patient-centred care skills' (Chambers and Ryder 2009). It is clear from this discussion that within the politics of nursing and health care, a values approach has been adopted and applied to policy, education and practice but without necessarily taking account of the potential emotional costs. Doctoral scholarship may offer opportunities to redress this balance.[19]

Emotional labour costs

As the following account from an interview with a student nurse in my first study testifies, patients and their families then, as now, valued and needed caring nurses. But these skills that Benner refers to as connection and involvement require both teaching and learning in order to protect the nurse and heal the patient.

I asked the student to describe any incidents that she had found particularly stressful during her training. She told me about her time on the paediatric ward when she became involved with a young child and her family.

> There just happened to be a patient on the paediatric ward at the time, a little girl who had cancer and for some reason she took to me. And in a good way and in a bad way I think this was encouraged because she loathed being in hospital. She was six.

Q. *How good and bad?*

She had a lot of chemotherapy and she died in the end, but it was good I think because she took to me, her mother did and her family did. But bad because it all became a bit too much really.

Q. *In what way too much?*

Well stressful really. I didn't say at work but I should have done. It was silly of me because there is a very highly esteemed teacher up there and I am sure she would have been very helpful now I think about it. But at the time you want to look as though you're coping. I mean the trained staff are there but they all knew that this child had taken to me so much and I was obviously being very useful to her making hospital not quite perhaps so unbearable as it had been, but it was quite a strain. I think it was from her mother more than her. Obviously her mother was very anxious.

I'm surprised nobody actually said to me 'are you managing, is it alright?' I think they forget about that side of nursing. They think 'Oh yeah, you're a nurse, you can manage'. But you can't really. I mean we're still pretty young. Outwardly you might be managing, but you know I used to go home and cry my eyes out sometimes. It was dreadful. But I've found that at work well you've almost got to be, well people expect you to be happy and not cross. And you can't be cross even though you feel like wringing someone's neck! You've got to be reasonably under control and of course everybody suffers when you go home.

I think you learn to stop that, you learn to switch off and be different, forget about work when you go home, I mean you've got to.

Q. *And do you think you learn that?*

I think you do, but through trial and error.

First, the student recognizes the importance of giving emotional support to a child and her family and the need for 'connection and involvement'. But she also describes how she was pulled down by her lack of skill in handling her involvement in the absence of trained staff, who recognized and supported the emotional cost of caring. She recognizes that, as a nurse, she is expected to be happy rather than cross and expected to manage and cope with extremes of feelings. As these expectations come from her seniors, she consequently expects them of herself. Like Hochschild's flight attendants, she must induce or suppress her own feelings, some would say subordinate them, to make others feel cared for and safe, irrespective of how she feels herself. She learns through 'trial and error' to 'switch off' and 'forget about work' when she goes home. But is this through surface acting to the point that she can no longer remain involved with patients other than at a superficial level, at risk of becoming detached and alienated? Or can she learn through experience and systematic training to recognize and use her feelings to remain therapeutically involved both for herself and the patient?

Hochschild's findings suggest that she can. One group of flight attendants that she studied received intensive training in the use of deep and surface acting to manage their emotions in given situations. Older, more experienced workers were found to be particularly adept at deep acting which allowed them to distinguish between their 'personal' and 'work' selves, develop a 'healthy' estrangement between self and work role and prevent burn out.

The acting techniques employed by the flight attendants seem feasible for the duration of a flight, but nurses have to sustain emotional involvement for much longer periods. Often they develop their own emotional labour strategies,[20] some of which are positive, but many of which evolve to protect them from a range of feelings: guilt, fear, failure and anger, to name a few.

How do Hochschild's notions of deep and surface acting apply to nurses' accounts of their presentation of self to the outside world?

Hochschild's suggestion that we manage our emotions according to feeling rules represented, for me, a framework for interpreting the empirical reality I encountered through the students' accounts and my own field observations. The students quoted above clearly appeared to be managing their feelings, whether it was to carry on as if nothing had happened when a patient had shouted or been rude to them, or to make a little girl's stay in hospital not seem quite so unbearable, despite feeling personally upset by her condition.

An account from 1998 shows that student nurses continued to feel vulnerable to what can be interpreted as the emotional insensitivities of qualified staff. The following vignette was brought to my attention by a colleague during a debriefing session following student placements. The vignette again concerned a student's experience on a paediatric ward. The student had been very unhappy during her placement, and her colleagues had encouraged her to describe her experience to their lecturer. The student had become involved with a young patient, bringing her presents and kind words. The ward staff had criticized her for her involvement with this patient and suggested this was not a good way to begin her nursing career. Indeed there was even a suggestion that she may not be a suitable candidate to be a nurse at all.

The lecturer talked through the situation with the student and discovered that she had been hospitalized as a child herself. They agreed that her history could account for her need to care for the young patient because she was symbolically caring for her childhood self. The student was reassured that her reactions were quite 'normal' and that far from being unsuitable for a nursing career, her obvious sensitivity and empathy for the child were future qualities she could draw on. The incident also demonstrated the importance of skilled mentoring on the part of the lecturer to encourage and support the student's emotional insights and subsequent capacity for emotional labour (Williams 1999).

A mature approach to supporting students to care for young patients in emotionally difficult situations is illustrated by the following account which was described by a concerned social worker. It also offers a more optimistic view of how students can be supported in the future.

A child branch nursing student at the end of her second year was asked to sit with a seriously ill boy suffering from cancer. His father was also sitting with him and was extremely distressed by his son's obvious extreme pain. The student went to tell her mentor that she was concerned at the boy's distress and wondered whether he could be given further analgesia. The mentor told her to 'hang on in there' that the pain the boy was experiencing was not unusual and would settle down with soothing words. This was not the case, and the boy's father told the student that he was convinced something 'different' was happening. After two further conversations with her mentor, the student finally persuaded her to take the situation seriously. On investigating the cause of the boy's distress, the mentor discovered that the extreme pain was indeed 'different' from prior symptoms and caused by a pathological fracture of the femur. Appropriate action was taken, and the student and the boy's father dissolved into tears of relief that something was finally being done but concerned that a fracture had been discovered.

This was not the end of the story. Once appropriate action had been taken to relieve the boy's pain, the mentor sat down with the student to discuss what had taken place. First of all she apologized for not having taken the student's first report seriously and admitted that this was partly because she had been busy and preoccupied with another patient. She also reflected on the importance of her own need to actively listen to both frontline carers and relatives and take their concerns seriously and immediately. When the student admitted she would rather not have cried in front of the patient and his father, the mentor comforted her and suggested that sometimes such obvious concern can be appreciated by patients and their relatives and friends. She also noted that if the mentor had taken heed of the student when she first reported her concern about the boy, then she may not have been reduced to public tears.

This account is heartening because it demonstrates the key role the mentor can play in supporting students to care and the ability of this particular mentor to be self critical. It also bears out one leader's view that:

> The qualified accountable nurse as mentor is much more important than the Ward Sister in showing that learning is done. They are responsible for their students' learning.

However, the account also demonstrates the dual demands on mentors to deliver a service as well as teach and supervise students. As this mentor was well aware, teaching students was seen as taking second place to delivering patient care.

The patients in these accounts were the recipients of the students' emotional labour who in turn were supported either by each other or their mentors. But what did patients expect of nurses and how did their expectations contribute to the feeling rules that shaped their relationships with them?

Everybody's ideal

In 1984, when I asked patients to describe a 'good' nurse they were more likely to talk about attitudes and feelings rather than technical competence.

Forty-four different words or phrases were used by the patients to describe 'ideal' and 'real' nurses. Only six of these words or phrases referred to functional rather than to affective attributes. Coser (1962), who designed the original interview agenda (see: Companion website, Methodological Appendix I, Smith 1992), reported similar findings. Words used to describe nurses' functional attributes included efficient, observant, alert and 'capable of doing their job'. One patient combined both functional and affective attributes by expecting nurses to be 'caring but efficient'. As we shall see in Chapter 5, ward sisters also distinguished between nurses' functional and affective attributes. The caring (i.e. emotional) aspects of nursing were clearly seen as distinct but complementary to and underpinning the functional (i.e. efficient, observant, capable, alert) aspects.

Kindness, helpfulness and patience were the affective or caring aspects most frequently used to describe the City Hospital nurses. Nurses were said to keep patients happy by being cheerful, loving, considerate, friendly and understanding and made them feel at home. Talking, listening, showing interest and sympathy featured as examples of the ideal nurse. As one patient concluded:

> A nurse has to be aware of the patient's condition and how to tackle it. She has to have a nursing manner which requires a lot of patience and forethought and to try and relieve pain and suffering not by medical means but by compassion.

This quotation is interesting because the patient has a clear view that a nursing manner requires patience, forethought and compassion to relieve pain and suffering, which are distinct from medical means.

In a contemporary study, service users with long-term physical or mental health conditions and their carers emphasized that good communication promoted positive feelings of being in control and being valued, and were at the top of their list when evaluating the quality of their care (Ross et al. 2009). As one respondent said speaking for others, 'If I know what is going on I feel more positive and in control', while another respondent was grateful to staff who showed 'the time or willingness to listen to my concerns'. When asked what would make care better one respondent said: 'putting people first' or 'treating patients as individuals' and 'with dignity'. Once more the little things emerged as important, and those professionals who 'went beyond their remit' and ensured that the little things don't 'get forgotten' were very much appreciated.

The nurse as emotional labourer

From the 1980s data it emerged that patients, like students, realized that nurses had to work emotionally on themselves in order to care for patients. This view of care as emotional labour suggests that, potentially, patients recognize that caring is more than just part of the package of women's work.

The following quotations offer some interesting perspectives on the nurse as emotional labourer.

The first patient, a young man in his thirties, was a trained laboratory technician. He had had a lot of hospital experience, both as a worker and patient, and had even been a student nurse for a brief period. His background and interests therefore gave him some interesting insights. He said:

> As a nurse you are more at the beck and call of the public than in a supermarket. I tell the nurse don't forget you're only human. You see them when the patient keeps ringing the bell and they grimace to themselves. Then they go up to the patient all smiles.

Here he compared the nurse with another service sector worker, the supermarket assistant. The difference between the two, he believed, was that the nurse was more vulnerable to the demands of the public. He closely observed the reaction of the nurse to the 'demanding' patient who kept on ringing his call bell for assistance. She grimaced, irritated that yet again she was being called. But she couldn't show the patient she was irritated; so she transformed her grimace into smiles as she approached him. The patient who was recounting this story clearly recognized that this transformation cost 'superhuman' effort by reminding the nurses that they were only human.

The second patient was also in his thirties and had had multiple hospital admissions for a chronic condition. As I spoke to him he implied he had been hurt by getting too close to nurses in the past. He valued those nurses who made him feel at home, but he was also aware that 'care can be dangerous if you are emotional about patients, you can't let it affect you, it's got to be platonic'. The view that being emotional was dangerous and that platonic care was preferable is interesting in the light of an analysis of emotional labour. The importance of making the patient feel that care is safe rather than dangerous again shows that managing emotions requires skill over and above 'natural' caring qualities, and is different from love.

Patients, like students, identified caring as the emotional side of nursing as being distinct but complementary to and underpinning the functional (efficient, observant, capable, alert) attributes of the 'ideal' nurse. Some patients recognized that nurses had to work emotionally on themselves (undertake emotional labour) in order to appear caring at all times. This observation is of immense importance, because it potentially recognizes that caring is more than just part of the package of women's work and requires specialist learning to produce in others a sense of feeling cared for in a safe place.

In the 2000s the increase in the patient population with complex long-term conditions living at home and the changes in service provision to respond to their needs resulted in community staff feeling stressed and emotional and pushed to the limit by their perceptions that patient safety was being put at risk (Ross et al. 2009, Smith et al. 2009).

Hochschild (1989) also looked at work in the home by focusing on the emotional life of two job couples and the different strategies adopted by working parents for dividing domestic labour and gratitude in the home. She showed how gender ideologies may either reinforce or conflict with reality. Feeling rules came into play, which guided emotion work to produce a gender-specific strategy to cope with the conflict. Hochschild concluded that one of the most important costs to women is that society devalues the work of the home and sees women as inferior because they do devalued work. Professional care work undertaken in the home may be similarly devalued.

What then are the implications of these findings for nurses, given that nursing reproduces many of the traditional female roles and domestic tasks in the workplace? What is the fit between gender and occupational ideologies? Do conflicts arise and if so what feelings are generated? Do feeling rules come into play to guide emotion work and produce strategies to cope with these conflicts? If so, how do they manifest themselves? And how does the gender dimension of care shaped by twenty-first century changes in service delivery continue to be an important factor in the emotional labour of nursing?

In the seven chapters that follow, I comment on my original 1980s research, re-examine some of these questions and ask others in relation to nurses as emotional labourers. I present new research data to address these questions as well as the key question: can nurses still care? The original material was used to construct a series of close-up portraits, nurses' own accounts and reflections on the nature of nursing and caring. Each chapter progresses to examine the viability of emotional labour as a concept: nurses' different emotional styles; the students' training trajectories and how they learn to care; the role of the ward sister in setting the emotional tone; the legitimization of emotional labour and the forms it takes between both nurses and nurses on the one hand and nurses and patients on the other; the strategies nurses adopt both to keep in touch and protect themselves from their feelings. New theoretical perspectives and empirical data are drawn upon to interrogate the original data and offer new insights to student nurses' experiences of learning nursing and caring.

Perspectives were offered in my first book on the content and structure of nurse training that was judged to be relevant to planning and implementing Project 2000. Since then the new 'Fitness for Practice' curriculum has been implemented following critiques of Project 2000, and new data that investigated contemporary students' experience of learning in the current educational and clinical climate have been drawn upon (Allan et al. 2008a). The Nursing and Midwifery Council (NMC) has been in consultation with the nursing profession on current educational provision in order to revise the curriculum in readiness for the new graduate level programmes required for 2013 (NMC 2010a, 2010b). Furthermore, the political landscape is on the brink of change as the coalition government established in May 2010 draws up radical plans following a major spending review to cut back public sector investment. Traditionally, nursing has fared badly during economic downturns revealing the susceptibility of the female workforce to market forces.

In summary then, this second book focuses on nurses and nursing as portrayed through contemporary popular and professional rhetoric to re-examine the notion of emotional labour as a component of caring, how nurses care and learn to care and its effects on carers and the cared for. Since the publication of the first book in 1992, many other research studies have been undertaken which add new perspectives on the emotional labour analysis, and some of these studies have already been highlighted in this chapter. The external global, policy and educational changes that have taken place in the intervening years will also form part of the analysis in seeking to understand the changing contexts in which nurses work, learn and care.

Putting their toe in the water: selecting, testing and expecting nurses to care

Research subjects, settings and methods

The 1984 study

I began my first study in 1984 as the demographic time bomb and the nursing recruitment crisis began to challenge the assumption that there would always be an unlimited supply of young women motivated to become nurses.[1]

The setting for the research was a typical British teaching hospital where, as one study showed, most of the direct nursing (about 75 per cent) was provided by nurses in training (Moores and Moult 1979). These nurses were usually between 18 and 21 years old and faced a range of life and death issues in the prime of their lives.

In order to gather data and gain insights into the research setting I worked as a nurse in a number of wards and attended classes in the school of nursing. In this way I was able to re-experience the world of the student nurse and to construct their three-year training trajectories (see: Companion website, Appendix A, Smith 1992). I also conducted in-depth interviews with nurses and patients.

In addition I distributed over 500 student questionnaires on the ward learning environment. The questionnaire, developed and tested by Joan Fretwell (1985), was based on her research in nurse training schools and gave me very useful complementary information. It enabled me to cover a much wider population of students and wards beyond the subjects of my in-depth study (see: Companion website, Methodological Appendix I, Smith 1992).

This first study took place at a unique moment in the history of nurse education i.e. on the eve of the introduction of the Project 2000 curriculum and the demise of apprenticeship-style training, a style that had essentially been in operation since Nightingale's time. I combined ethnography and grounded theory in a case study of a traditional nursing school, the 'City' Hospital, described in its nurse recruitment brochures, and by patients, as 'Friendly and welcoming'. 'The City Nurse' was identified as the ideal nurse who was technically competent, caring and efficient, and 'looked like a model'.

The nursing school and hospital were part of the same organization i.e. the National Health Service (NHS), and the students were the main workforce, and as one student observed, student nurses as a group 'care more, because there are more of us'. The City Hospital nurse managers were clear that patient care should be undertaken by students supervised by ward sisters, and they saw no place for the employment of nursing auxiliaries to replace student labour. At the time commentators put this attitude down to the class nature of nursing at City Hospital, resulting in a workforce that was predominantly young white middleclass and female. Nursing auxiliaries employed elsewhere throughout the NHS were more likely to be older, mature women and men from working class and Black and Ethnic Minority (BME) backgrounds.

The need for a new study in the 2000s

The structure of the health service and the organization of nurse education have completely changed since the original study was undertaken in the 1980s. Students now follow a three-year university education to study for either a diploma or degree rather than for a hospital-based certificate. A pilot study in the late 1990s revealed that at the level of the ward, the role of the ward sister had changed and that the mentor had become the person responsible for the student's day-to-day learning as well as patient care (Smith and Gray 2001a, 2001b).

The pilot study[2] was extended in 2006 to find out more about these changes as well as the content and process of student nurse learning and the status of care and emotions in the new NHS (Allan et al. 2008a). The study began with senior educators in professional and statutory bodies and four case study universities who were interviewed to obtain their views on the current status of nursing and nurse education.

Twenty years ago, at the time of the original study, it was easy to locate a discrete case study based on a local hospital school of nursing where the students were an integral part of the hospital workforce. Now students' primary base is at a university with placements likely to be at some distance away in a variety of NHS trusts. In the subsequent study, sampling methods and selection of clinical case studies were set up to reflect the modern day organization and control of nurse education.

A modified version of the original ward learning environment questionnaire[3] was sent on-line to all students in the four case study universities who were currently on placement in order to access a wide range of respondents at different stages of training and in different specialities backed up by 12 episodes of in-depth observation in acute clinical areas and interviews with students and staff involved in teaching and learning (see: Companion website, Methodological Appendix I, Smith 1992, and Methodological Appendix II, Smith 2012).

Who train as nurses?

1984–1985

The nursing workforce at 'City' Hospital[4] was typical of most teaching hospitals in the 1980s. By far the largest group comprised the trainee nurses, aged between 18 and 21, on the frontline of patient care. They also best fitted the public image of the nurse as 'young lady' or 'good woman' and Nightingale's descendant who was vocationally motivated, obedient and subservient to both medical and nursing superiors.

To what extent this image of the nurse was ever an accurate or representative perception is open to speculation since historically the nursing workforce in Britain has not been a homogeneous group (Bellaby and Oribabor 1980). Their class, gender and racial composition may vary according to grade, speciality, institution or region in which they work. But the predominant image of the nurse as white, middle-class and female prevailed and affected the content of their work, training, and public and professional expectations and prospects.[5]

2006–2008

The predominant image of nurses as white, middle class and female is no longer necessarily the case. The results of the questionnaire survey gave some indication of who train as nurses in the modern NHS. When the survey sample was checked against the national statistics for 2006 it appeared to be broadly similar to the student nurse population in UK Universities.

Ward learning environment questionnaire respondents

Demographic characteristics

Over half the respondents (59%) were mature students (26 years and over) while less than a half (41%) were under 26 years old. The gender dimension remained largely unchanged: 89% of respondents were female compared with only 11% male. Over two-thirds of the students i.e. 68% described their ethnicity as White or White British, the next largest ethnic group was African (9%), followed by Black or Black British (7%). Just over half the respondents described themselves as single rather than married or living with a partner. Sixty per cent of the respondents did not have any children while 40% had at least one child.

Educational qualifications

At the time of the first study students' educational qualifications at the City Hospital tended to be higher than that of the national average because as a teaching hospital there was an expectation that the students would have studied for the Advanced Level General Certificate of Education (A Levels). The educational qualifications of the on-line survey respondents in 2006 reflected the move of nursing into higher education in that nearly one in five respondents (18%) was already a graduate; a very small proportion (2%) had a Master's degree and one respondent had a PhD. Nearly half (48%) had A Levels. Almost a fifth (19%) had the General Certificate of Secondary Education or the Ordinary Level General Certificate of Education (GCSEs / O Levels) while 13% had at least one General National Vocational Qualification (GNVQ). Those students with A Levels or a degree were much more likely to be studying for a nursing degree than a diploma.

Programme and year of study

Eighty-three per cent of respondents were studying for a nursing diploma, and the remaining 17% were studying for a degree. Ninety-six per cent of respondents were studying full-time; just 4% were studying part-time. Over three-quarters of the respondents (77%) were undertaking the adult nursing programme, 14 % were mental health nursing students, 9% were child health students with just two students (less than 1%) in the learning disability branch. The largest group of respondents (45%) was in their second year, followed by 29% in their third year and 26% in their first year.

Comparisons with the Nursing and Midwifery Admissions Service (NMAS) National Data Base for 2006 (NMAS 2007) suggest my sample was similar in that the majority of students were studying adult nursing. Their gender composition was also similar but they were rather more mature and ethnically diverse. They were also much more likely to be studying for a diploma than suggested by the national statistics (HESA 2004/05). This could have been because students in their first and second years who registered for the diploma at the time of the survey may have converted to the degree programme in their third year, but their final qualification at registration would not have shown up in the analysis.[6]

'Too posh to wash'

The 'dis-ease' with which nurses and nursing assume the academic mantel and the dissonance with which it is viewed in the public discourse is no more apparent in the 'too posh to wash' lobby which discredited the Project 2000 initiative and began the educational review that resulted in the 'Fitness for Practice' curriculum in 1999 (UKCC 1999, NMC 2004a). Scott (2004) notes that the lobby was underpinned by accusations that the move of student nurses into universities had rendered them 'too posh to wash' resulting in a general lowering of standards, including poor hygiene and outbreaks of serious infection. Issues of recruitment and retention changed in the intervening years from the luxury of being able to preserve a homogeneous workforce to concerns for meeting workforce targets set by the Department of Health as part of the government's plan for the New NHS and the response of the Strategic Health Authorities to supply an appropriately educated workforce.

The announcement that nursing is set to become an all-graduate profession from 2013 has reignited the 'too posh to wash' debate. Nursing leaders are clear that the change is 'right' for the profession. As the Chief Nurse for England pointed out 'More young people than ever are studying for a degree and this will make nursing more attractive to them' (cited on whitehallpages. net, http://www.whitehallpages.net 2009). The Prime Minister's Commission on Nursing and Midwifery, which reported just weeks before the 2010 General Election, recommended that degree level study was essential to the development of nurses' decision-making skills in 'the transformed NHS' (Prime Minister's Commission 2010). Although a change in government makes the report's future uncertain, the 20 high-profile nursing and midwifery leaders who were members of the Commission are unlikely to let one of their key recommendations go. For the Chief Executive of the Nursing and Midwifery Council (NMC) new graduate programmes are required to produce competent nurses able to combine 'basic' and 'complex' care and 'provide higher quality for all'. A similar view was expressed by the Royal College of Nursing's (RCN) secretary general, who said 'Many nursing roles are demanding and involve increasingly advanced levels of practice and clinical knowledge'. These nursing leaders clearly see the need for nurses and midwives to work in new and complex ways supported by advanced levels of knowledge and skills. But the perennial question continues to trouble both public and professionals alike: 'does equipping nurses with technical and academic expertise, render them less compassionate and able to care?'

In a feature clearly targeted at addressing this critique a number of opinion setters from the Department of Health, the NMC, the RCN, the trade unions and the professionals themselves, clearly think not. The majority continue to challenge the 'too posh to wash' argument with a clear message that safe compassionate care and academic achievements are not 'mutually exclusive' (www. publicservice.co.uk, 1 April 2010). Nursing is still a predominantly female profession in that the persistence of the debate is clearly linked to gender. One commentator observed that other health professionals educated to degree level do not get 'tarred with the same brush' while another commented that the public would be unlikely to react so strongly to all graduate entry 'if the nursing profession was overwhelmingly male'. Nursing and caring are still perceived to be inextricably linked to personal rather than professional skill and academic qualifications to detract from nurses' ability or motivation to care. A specialist nurse countered this argument by asserting that 'academic knowledge' enables specialist nursing teams 'to identify and deliver the best possible care for their patients'. These public dialogues reveal that there is still a need to recognize, analyze and value care as well as to counter the argument that a graduate education will militate against the nurse's capacity to care. Emotional labour as a conceptual device with the potential to link caring and learning remains as relevant today as when I first discovered it over two decades ago.

Recruitment and retention

In 1983 nurse managers and educators in charge of recruitment at City Hospital were able to maintain the student workforce not only in the image of Nightingale i.e. white, middle-class and female but also an individual who had a credible academic background. How did they do this?

The job prospectus

One way of maintaining the image was through the job prospectus. The first page read:

> It is the aim of the hospital to create a friendly and happy atmosphere in which nurses can more easily care for the physical and psychological needs of the patient and fulfil their desire to be of service to others.

Of interest here is the commitment to the creation of a friendly and happy atmosphere, but also that such an atmosphere facilitates caring. Caring is clearly identified as what nurses do, but more importantly it is underpinned by the assumption

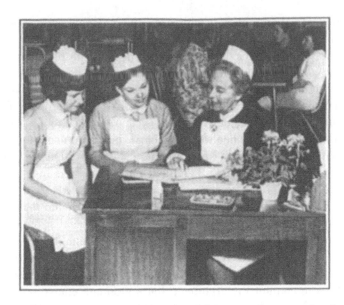

Illustration 2.1   Recruitment images at the beginning of the research portrayed student nurses and ward sisters as white and female
Source: Hospital Recruitment Brochure. Reproduced with kind permission.

that caring *fulfils* a nurse's *desire* to be of *service* to others. Like Hochschild's applicants to become flight attendants, prospective nurses were being introduced to the 'rules of the game' through the language of the prospectus, even before interview.

The 'rules' were compounded by photographs contained in the prospectus which showed images of young white women engaged in a number of professional and personal activities: talking with patients and colleagues, studying in the library, playing tennis and dressmaking. Images of male and black nurses were noticeably absent. Recent versions of the prospectus, like the national recruitment campaigns, included such images. Recreational activities were more varied, and tennis and dressmaking had given way to cultural and culinary pursuits about town. The new prospectus, however, retained much of the language of the earlier version promoting nursing as care and concern.

In the 2000s the recruitment images are portrayed on national and individual university websites. Publicity material, such as glossy recruitment brochures portray smiling engaged nursing and midwifery students alongside other students from engineering, music and science. Most faculties, departments or schools of nursing may also produce their own specialist materials. Nurses are portrayed in a variety of settings whether in the high-tech environment of the high dependency unit or engaged in classroom discussion with fellow students. The theme is one of care and attention between nurses and their patients: they still touch, hold, smile

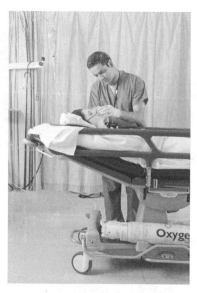

Illustration 2.2   In the high dependency unit: young man in 'scrubs'
Source: Thinkstock. Reproduced with kind permission.

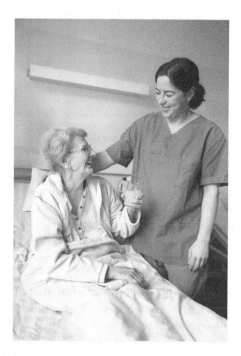

Illustration 2.3   Mature student in 'scrubs' in a medical ward
Source: iStockphoto. Reproduced with kind permission of iStockphoto.

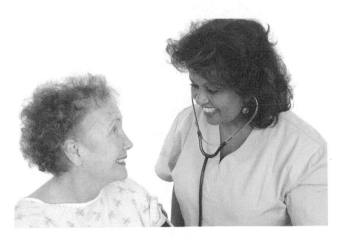

Illustration 2.4 A postgraduate nurse practitioner
Source: Thinkstock. Reproduced with kind permission.

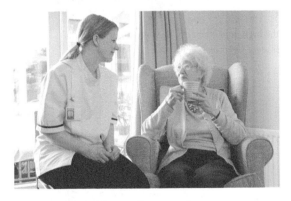

Illustration 2.5 Student reminisces with a care home resident
Source: Thinkstock. Reproduced with kind permission.

and perform technical tasks. The profile of the students reflects the diversity of the workforce whether from a BME background, a young man, a mature woman, mostly smiling but also serious, intense and engaged. One interesting feature to note in contemporary marketing and publicity materials is that 'scrubs' frequently replace the uniform dresses and tunics of the 1980s and 1990s in modern day nursing images as illustrated.

University websites also publish the results of national surveys, such as the National Student Survey and those conducted by national newspapers such as the *Guardian, Independent and the Times* especially to publicize high ratings. There is fierce competition to attract students to apply for their programmes, and Nursing is no exception. These conditions present a very different set of recruitment issues at the City Hospital School of 20 years ago, when nurse recruiters

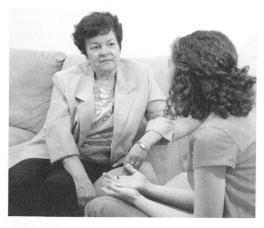

Illustration 2.6   Patient or compassionate counsellor?
Source: Thinkstock. Reproduced with kind permission.

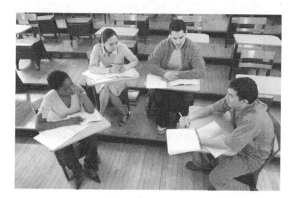

Illustration 2.7   Group work in the classroom
Source: Thinkstock. Reproduced with kind permission.

had the pick of a large pool of applicants for a relatively small number of places. Typically, there are now places available for up to two intakes of 300 diploma students and 70 degree students per year.

Selection procedures

1984–1985

City Hospital was popular among prospective student nurses, and six times the number of candidates applied annually to fill the 180 places available. Thus the

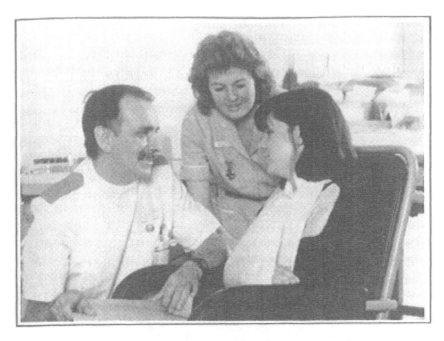

Illustration 2.8   In 1990s recruitment images, male and black nurses are no longer absent: staff nurse with student and patient

Source: Chris Priest. Reproduced with kind permission.

nurse recruiters found themselves with a large pool of applicants from which they could select students judged to possess the necessary qualities, not only to become nurses, but more specifically to train at City.

These qualities included working with people and academic ability, as measured by obtaining Ordinary Level passes in the General Certificate of Education. Candidates were expected to have obtained a minimum of five Ordinary Level passes.

Nurse recruiters at City, in line with most teaching hospitals, not only looked for 'personal' qualities in their candidates but also for a higher educational standard than the national entry requirements of two Ordinary Level passes.[7]

During interviews, I began to note how the two types of selection criteria presented students with seemingly contradictory versions of nursing. On the one hand, they were selected because of their interest in and experience of working with people. On the other, they were expected to have reached a good educational standard with priority being given to those students who had obtained passes in biological subjects. An analysis of the students' entry qualifications showed that the majority of them had obtained an Ordinary Level pass in biology, and almost a third of them had also obtained an Advanced Level pass in the subject. The

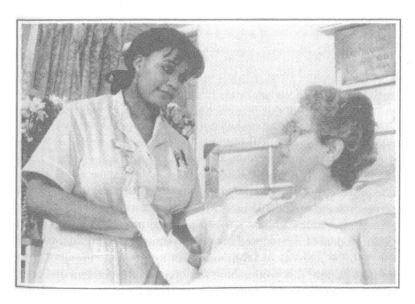

Illustration 2.9   Student nurse with patient
Source: Chris Priest. Reproduced with kind permission.

number of people with passes in socially orientated subjects, such as history and sociology, was much lower.

The differences in defining the two types of selection criteria implied that a student's interest and experience in working with people came as part of the personal and experiential package that they brought with them as vocationally orientated young women, whereas the biological knowledge required to nurse had to be learnt formally and validated both before and during training.

A patient who was a public relations officer and interested in recruitment issues told me that compared to other hospitals she'd been in, there was something 'special' about the City Hospital. She continued:

> In my independent view it's because of the selection. The nurses are all on an even keel. They've always a smile, always got time for you and make you feel as if you're a person and not just passing through.

This patient's comment was interesting because she was essentially describing the behavioural characteristics of the City nurse as emotional labourer ('on an *even* keel', 'always a smile', 'always got time for you') which made her feel cared for (being made to feel like a person; 'not just passing through'). Her reference to selection confirmed the recruiter's view that selecting nurses who had already put their toe in the water with the general public ensured that they were more likely to maintain outward composure, even with patients who were not being nice.

2006–2008

Nowadays, universities are subject to commissioned targets from their Strategic Health Authorities and therefore are under pressure to fill funded places for degrees and diplomas. Student selection is usually based on open days, interviews and academic achievements and low recruitment results in loss of income and ultimately teaching staff to balance the books. In 2011, as this book goes to press, student numbers, clinical nursing and teaching posts are coming under scrutiny as part of a major government spending review.

In the follow-up study it was possible to capture some of the reasons why students decided to become nurses. It was also possible to get a sense of the demographic characteristics of those students both willing and available to be interviewed to provide a snapshot of the student nurse population more generally. For example, of the eleven students I interviewed in one university, four were in the 18–21 year age group, and the majority of seven were 'mature' students in their thirties, forties and fifties. Within this group, there was one male respondent and one person from a BME group. Three students were studying for a Bachelor's degree, one student was undertaking a Master's degree and seven students were studying for the diploma. Most of the students had worked as volunteers or had been in paid 'people' work prior to beginning their formal nurse education. The most common previous employment was as an HCA, often in a nursing or care home, but also included other types of 'people work' such as banking and hospitality.

A focus group discussion with three 'mature' participants describes why they decided to become student nurses. Two had worked as HCAs and one had worked in a bank. The HCAs had particularly wanted to undertake their nurse training because they felt there was only so far they could go even with National Vocational Qualification (NVQ) training level 3 'when you couldn't even give an aspirin'. They all agreed nursing had to be 'something you want to do; you've got to love the job' because 'it's not an easy thing to do. You don't get a lot of thanks or money'. All of them had taken a drop in salary to become student nurses.

One student described doing double shifts as 'hard work' for which 'there has to be something pushing you' to which another student added 'a good nurse is prepared to go that extra mile for nothing'.

They also thought that having had other life experiences before coming into nursing was very important and all agreed that:

> Not everyone can do it (nursing). It's got to be something you want to do. Life experience gives you commonsense, which if you come straight from school you don't have. You don't have that knowledge of how to speak to patients.

They described their student cohort of 35 students who, during the course of their three-year training, had had close to a 50 per cent attrition rate, leaving only 17 students to complete. Many of the leavers had been the 'younger ones who didn't know what they were going in for'. A project at one of the other sites to investigate why students left before completing training confirmed this observation that the highest attrition rates (26.9%) were in the 18–20 year age group. In the older age groups the attrition rates decreased with students over 41 years to around 12%.[8]

One of the participants had decided to become a nurse because of her experiences as a patient, which had highlighted the importance of good communication and the importance of being a good listener in order to make the hospital experience less traumatic. Her sensitivity to the importance of communication had also been highlighted by her previous experience in the customer service department of a large bank. She said:

> I want to care, be involved with caring for patients and help them to get through. They can be very scared, very vulnerable in a strange environment.

All three participants described their selection interviews as long and probing. The students also reported how their previous experiences of working with people as volunteers or in paid care work had been viewed positively by their interviewers because they saw it as being highly relevant in preparing for nurse training.

Similar motivations for becoming nurses were also apparent during interviews with the younger students (aged 18–21 years). For two students, exposure to illness of a parent motivated them to become nurses. One student explained:

> Mum was ill when I was a child so that's what prompted me to want to be a nurse ...
>
> The nurses were lovely with my Mum and she never had a bad word to say about them. I think I wanted to help others like they'd helped my Mum so, that was quite important.

Another observed:

> When I was younger my dad got ill and we were going to hospital all the time and we had District Nurses come in the house and I think since then really.

It appears that the desire to care is still a central reason for why these students decided to become nurses. They recognize that there are aspects of nursing that go beyond its monetary rewards and that it can be hard physical work. But there are also technical aspects to the work that need specific training that go beyond the scope of the HCA role and training. They also recognize that nursing work is enhanced by 'commonsense' knowledge associated with life experience and on-the-job learning which in turn better prepares the new recruit and reduces the risk of attrition.

So these findings suggest that contemporary student nurses are required not only to stand up in the culture of a specific hospital or Trust as in the past but are faced with the more recent NHS environment of targets and outcomes.

Standing up in the NHS environment

The accounts from 1984 and 2007 illustrate that nurses, patients and recruiters consistently identify nursing as 'people' work in which, as Hochschild suggests, communication and encounter are central.

In the first study I specifically began to understand that students' emotional activities in which communication and encounter are central, were controlled by the regular practical assessments conducted during their ward placements. These assessments, like Hochschild's third characteristic of emotional labour jobs, provided a mechanism to allow the employer, in this case the students' senior nurses and teachers, to exercise a degree of control over their emotional activities by regularly assessing them on their personal and professional qualities.

Although I described assessment procedures in operation at the City Hospital, all schools of nursing were required by the training inspectorate[9] to operate similar systems. We can assume, therefore, that an analysis of systems at other schools would yield similar general findings.

The methods by which the students were tested at City were described in their plan of training as a 'series of structured and informal assessments based on detailed objectives' and 'a means by which encouragement is given to learners to *reach and maintain a high standard of nursing care throughout training*' (my emphasis). In other words, students were constantly under pressure to perform well.

The content of the assessments reflected the qualities for which the students had been selected, namely their ability to stand up in an environment that was friendly, hierarchical and academically demanding.

The detailed learning objectives for the general ward placements were concerned with acquiring competence in techniques and procedures associated with the care of patients suffering from specific diseases. Thus the assessment of the student's clinical learning was based on the view of their recruiters, that an academically demanding environment required them to understand clinical medicine. Out of 35 general ward learning objectives, only two dealt with patients' psychosocial needs. On nine out of fifteen wards, students were formally assessed usually by the trained ward staff on a number of specific procedures such as aseptic technique and drug administration. Students were also assessed on nursing skills related to patient care and managing colleagues. By the time they had reached their third year, for example, they were expected to plan, organize and ensure quality of care given both by themselves and their colleagues.

Other criteria on which the nurses were assessed related more specifically to the personal qualities for which they had been selected. They included 'personal appearance', communication with patients and an awareness of cultural, spiritual, physical and psychological needs. Students were also expected to be able to prioritize care, ensure safety at all times, report and record care given, evaluate it in terms of its effects on patients, use teaching opportunities and evaluate their own performance. These personal criteria on which the students were judged in 1984 were reinforced by the format of their ward reports given to them at the end of every ward placement (see Companion web site, Appendix B, Smith 1992).

Thus the methods by which the students were assessed throughout training reinforced the selection criteria on which they had been recruited, set the emotional tone of their work and served to maintain the image of the City nurse.

As one student saw it, 'In this hospital there is a very definite attempt to make you change your character, well, mould you into a "City" type'. I asked her what she meant by a City 'type'. She then described one of the ward sisters:

She's everybody's ideal, really. She's so sophisticated, she always looks so calm, attractive and manages to get all the work done. She's very kind and considerate and yet she looks almost like a model.

Here was a description of the 'ideal' City nurse who was also the ideal emotional labourer. She maintained calm, was kind and considerate, but also competent in that she managed to get all the work done in time. Her physical appearance was important. Not only was she described as 'attractive' but almost like a 'model'.

Another student described the role played by the teachers in their assessments which reinforced the hierarchical nature of their relationships. She said, 'You've got to respect a position of authority, but you shouldn't be scared like thinking "Oh god! she's going to be writing something about me". I don't want to be feeling like that about the school for three years'.

One of the tutors accurately captured the student's feelings when she said, 'they see us as their judge and jury'.

Another student experienced the ward reports as a way in which those in authority imposed a 'picture' or image of how they saw her. For her, 'the ward reports give you a picture of what they think you were like; not like I think I am'. She too said that confidence was the key quality on which the students were judged. 'It all depends on how confident you are. That's all they're interested in – "confidence"'.

But the first student added a rider which suggested that there was a fine balance between appearing confident and 'cocky' and that she found the staff's expectations difficult to interpret. 'I think it's quite difficult to see how they want you to behave as they don't want you to be "cocky"'. What she seemed to be describing here was the difference between the confidence expected of a 'young lady' able to stand up in a hierarchically demanding environment and the 'cocky' nurse able to stand up *for herself.* A nurse was expected to have the confidence to carry out complex orders and procedures, but rarely to question and never to answer back. In other words she learnt through being regularly assessed what was expected of her as a City nurse.

The negative feelings generated by this process were graphically described by two nurses nearing the end of their training. One nurse experienced the ward reports as 'a lot of character bashing'. The other felt that her identity had been crushed.

Yet all these students, whether they felt they were being moulded, seen in a different way to how they saw themselves, having their character bashed or their identity crushed, managed their private feelings in order to behave in the way expected of a City Hospital nurse. The methods by which the students were assessed therefore imposed feeling rules that required emotion work to maintain the image of the City nurse and trained them to stand up in a hierarchical and academically demanding environment.

One tutor observed:

> A problem may arise on the ward and the student might get unhappy but they won't say anything to the ward staff because they're frightened of the ward reports.

One student now at the end of training saw the assessments in a more positive and less passive light. She told me that through them she had built up both her confidence and role expectations and in the process learnt from other students to stick up for herself. She said:

> You don't think you'll have the confidence and be supportive and help and teach other students. But you build up to teaching and management responsibility through your assessments and you learn from other students to stick up for yourself.

Students in the 2000s gave similar but also distinctive views about their experiences of assessment and the central role played by their mentor in this process. Because they are no longer officially part of the workforce as salaried employees but supernumerary students, they have to be monitored and controlled in different ways than in the past when they were under the direct jurisdiction of the ward sister (Davies 1976). The students therefore have detailed paperwork to record the outcomes of their placements at different points over a four- to nine-week period.

During interviews with nurse educators, qualities such as personal appearance, punctuality and general attitude towards ward work were still identified as indicators of students' suitability to be nurses. There were even suggestions that supernumerary status and university education had undermined these qualities in the students. As one practice educator said:

> When the students are on their placements we have to ask the managers to oversee that they turn up at the appropriate time that they're wearing the appropriate gear,

because we have had people turn up in ripped jeans when they're working in clinical areas!

Another practice educator expressed particular concern about degree students. She said:

There's a more laissez faire attitude with the degree students if they're a bit late for their placements. It's no big deal for them, because that's the culture of University, isn't it? I think that knocks into nursing when they come into the ward area whereas we're like 'time keeping's important because the ward manager doesn't want to hand over twice'.

However they agreed that this attitude was not always dominant. One Practice Educator (PE) mentioned a second year student who stood out for her caring qualities to the extent that she 'outshone everyone even the trained staff'. Being caring was seen as the highest accolade.

But the language of care was absent in the type of paperwork current in nurse education which showed an expectation that students would become 'critical thinkers' and safe practitioners. In their 'Guide to Assessment of Practice' students were advised that:

The assessment of practice is a vital part of your course. You will gradually demonstrate an increasing development in:

- critical awareness
- reflective practice
- rational decision making
- clinical judgement

The students were then required throughout their three-year training to gather evidence to demonstrate achievement and development of practice which they could then store in the appropriate section of their Portfolio. They were also given guidelines by which to measure their progress against three levels of 'developing competence' during each year of their programme from Year 1 – 'Safe Practitioner' to Year 2 – 'Emerging Practitioner' and finally by the end of Year 3 to become an 'Effective Practitioner'. In addition their portfolio contained guidelines for each practice placement on how to use them.

One student explained how the system was intended to work but could break down if there were insufficient mentors and/or if they were not motivated to support them:

Sometimes there were too many students and not enough mentors, to fill in all your paperwork and you're worried about that, because they've got no time for you.

Another student explained the process:

You have an initial meeting where you set out your action plan, what you want to achieve from this ward.,, That's supposed to happen in the first week of your placement and then in the middle you're supposed to have to sit down with your mentor and they fill your paperwork in. Then your final meeting, you've got all these outcomes to fill in. You've got to write how you've achieved them. Then your mentor's supposed to go through and sign off that you've achieved them, and say whether you've passed your placement or not.

Methods of testing and assessment to ensure students are 'up to standard'

In the original study, methods of testing and assessing the students were in place in order to ensure that students were up to the standard expected of the City Hospital. In the current study, methods of testing and assessing work-based learning were set against national guidelines laid down by the NMC and implemented by the educational establishments where the students were registered. The role of the mentor/assessor and what was to be expected of the students during placements was specified in their documentation.

The role of the mentor/assessor

Typical documentation required the mentor/assessor to:

- prepare or update introductory materials in advance of the student's arrival;
- arrange a brief orientation programme to meet the team and acquaint the student with the working environment and resources, within the first week of placement;
- identify the learning needs with students;
- assist the student in developing an individual learning plan;
- provide a suitable learning environment in collaboration with other nurses and the multi-disciplinary team to support this plan;
- provide an objective, continuous assessment of the student's progress through regular, weekly supervision sessions and written comments in the report;
- liaise appropriately with clinical and academic teaching staff such as practice educators, clinical facilitators and link lecturers;
- complete an interim report on progress at the halfway point and a final written report at the end of the placement experience;
- make a final decision on the progress of the student and liaise with clinical or academic staff where appropriate and
- read and review the written evidence which supports the unit outcomes & sign them off as achieved.

Meeting with the mentor/assessor in practice to review progress

The students were reminded that they must be assessed, have their documentation 'signed off' by a qualified mentor and take responsibility for their learning. As the student describes above, this required them to meet their mentor at regular intervals during their placements to review their progress including three formal 'assessment' meetings: at the beginning to identify learning needs and opportunities; at the midway point to review progress and learning needs; and a final meeting to discuss overall performance and achievement of placement outcomes.

Mentor/assessor's assessment of and statement of achievement

The mentor/assessor's assessment of achievement was based on a combination of observation of the student's practice, discussion and the presentation of evidence. They would then be awarded a grade based on the following grading criteria:

S (successful) – the required criteria have been met

U (unsuccessful) – adequate opportunities have been provided but the required standard of achievement in meeting the specific unit outcomes/practice skills has not been reached

---

The criteria for success clearly laid the responsibility on the student rather than the mentor, with the inference being that it was up to the student to take advantage of these opportunities.

However, the current study revealed that some mentors found it hard to 'fail' students. Examples were given by PEs of students who had progressed through their three-year training only to be failed in their final placement necessitating them to take on a 'troubleshooting' role to deal with the situation. This finding was also apparent in a study undertaken by Duffy (NMC 2004b) for the NMC who reported that a 'failure to fail' students by mentors had become a common and worrying trend and that there was a need for more support from both education and practice to enable more effective assessment procedures to be put in place.

During a focus group discussion PEs showed similar concerns to those of Duffy's. For example one PE said:

> If a student needs to fail, which has happened on a couple of occasions, the mentors are usually reluctant to do it and it usually falls in my lap. So I tend to be just the trouble shooter.

Another PE agreed:

> Yes, people are too frightened to fail students and (to have a) confrontation, and I think that's why we come in more. I think that's more my role ... not necessarily failing students, but picking up on problem areas, because people don't like to do it; and we've just had a third year student who's failed her elective and has to redo the last part of her third year training. She was not safe to be in practice as a nurse and it was highlighted previously but nobody would fail her. Nobody wants to write bad things, do they?

A third PE added:

> You have to question why some of them are not picked up. We had one girl who ... was picked up on her second week. I had her in the office and I asked to speak to her, and it turned out when it got back to N at the University, that this was not the only ward that this had happened. N actually came to see us and said they were really worried about this student. But we were the only ward that had picked up the problems. Everybody else had passed the student ... It's unfair on the student as well as the staff, and they'd passed her on everything, when she shouldn't have been passed.

Clearly the mentors, despite the guidelines to do so, had not relayed their concerns to the PE. Duffy's recommendations were taken very seriously by the NMC with the result that a new system was put in place to set standards to support learning and assessment in practice and ascribe clear responsibility and accountability to a 'sign off mentor' i.e. a trained and named mentor who would 'sign off' a student's satisfactory level of competence at the end of each placement (NMC 2008a, NMC 2010c).

In the 1984 study I showed how the assessments controlled the students' behaviour whereas what seemed to be happening in 2007 was the other way round with the University through the student being perceived by the ward staff as being able to call the shots. However from the students' point of view, the university systems in place to monitor their placements and learning outcomes were highly dependent on their mentors for effective implementation. There were repeated examples during student interviews that this was a rather 'hit and miss' affair depending on the availability of the mentor and their recognition of and commitment to the role. As elaborated further in Chapter 5, the ability of mentors to perform their role depended effectively on the leadership, support and commitment of the ward manager. Furthermore, there was now an explicit expectation, not so apparent at the time of the first study, that students should take greater responsibility for their learning and become active learners, a feature I discuss further in Chapter 7.

In the first study students experienced a conflict of roles if their qualified colleagues acted as their assessors, or, as one tutor put it, they acted as their 'judge and jury'. Now this conflict of roles has become even more apparent as revealed by Bray and Nettleton (2007). They found that the role of mentor and assessor had become interchangeable, leading to confusion and conflict among both mentors and students.

For example one mentor said:

> I don't think people are 100% sure of what a mentor's role is and what they can and can't do and I think the difference between an assessor and a mentor, what is the difference? ... (Bray and Nettleton 2007, p. 853)

Students also used the term mentor and assessor interchangeably. The mentor/assessor was described as very busy with a range of commitments and insufficient time to complete the necessary paperwork. Consequently, their primary role and responsibility was perceived as student assessor and form filler rather than learning facilitator.

> I think the biggest issues really with mentors is time to fill in the forms ... Only two seemed to really understand your outcomes and help you to meet them. (Mentee 21 cited in Bray and Nettleton 2007, p. 853)

> Finding time to fill in the forms ... was stressful for myself and the assessors ... because of their commitments. (Mentee 26 cited in Bray and Nettleton 2007, p. 853)

Although the role of mentor as a leader for learning and assessment in clinical settings is clearly specified by the NMC (NMC 2008a) it remains an issue for further debate and discussion which I return to in Chapter 5.

In Nightingale's image

In the final section of this chapter, I examine the way in which the patients portrayed the City nurse in Nightingale's image and the students' reaction to this image. I then draw on new data to reassess that image in the context of current day nursing.

1980s style

In the first study, I observed a classroom discussion during which students were asked to describe the stereotypes patients had of them. They mentioned such images as 'angel', 'beautiful' and 'Florence Nightingale'.

I also found in my interviews with patients that the nurse as angel was a particularly popular image. One patient described a student as an 'angel of mercy' in the context of maintaining composure on a busy night shift when three elderly patients were shouting and confused and wandering up and down the ward. The

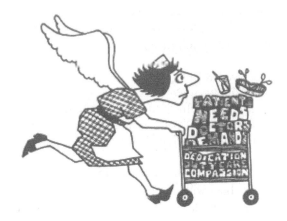

Illustration 2.10   1980s cartoon image of the nurse as 'angel'
Source: Cath Jackson. Reproduced with kind permission.

patient observed that the nurse was almost 'at breaking point and all white faced. I know I couldn't do it. It's hard to hold your temper. But she did very well to cope'. By inference her ability to 'hold her temper' was attributed to her being an 'angel of mercy'.

Associated with the image of the nurse as 'an angel' was also the belief by many patients that nursing was a 'vocation' which required dedication. One patient expressed surprise following discussions with some students because they told her that nursing was a 'job of work'. 'I'd always imagined it was a calling', she said.

The idea that nursing was a vocation epitomized the belief that nurses brought not only natural skills to their chosen occupation, but also deeper qualities of giving and lack of interest in financial reward. Two patients, for example, viewed nursing as something 'you've got to have in you'. Another patient saw nurse's abilities as 'resting so much on the girl, how much she can give to the patient. It goes with that nature that brings them into this sort of vocation'. Another patient reasoned that nursing must be a vocation since nurses 'wouldn't go in it for the money'. These images corresponded with those portrayed in the recruitment posters described in Chapter 1. Nurses had the essential qualifications before they went to school. They were also unlikely to be 'attracted to nursing because of the money'.

Nurses resented these images. One student told me that, 'patients call you an angel. I tell them I'm doing it not to go to heaven but as a job. They can't understand that'. A patient who was also a nurse challenged the image of the nurse as 'an angel of mercy'. Anyone can do it (nursing), she said, meaning that you didn't need to have a vocation to be a nurse.

These pictures suggest that, at the level of rhetoric, patients colluded in perpetuating the image of the nurse, a modern day Nightingale, as having 'natural' skills and being vocationally motivated and dedicated. Most students vigorously denied that they had been motivated by a vocation to choose nursing.

Perspectives for the 2000s

The 'too posh to wash' debates about the modern student nurse and the hostility expressed towards the decision to make nursing an all-graduate profession reflect the strong belief held by the public and others that becoming a nurse is vocationally motivated. These debates also beg the question 'Can nurses still care?' On the one hand recruiters are urged to improve their selection strategy, suggesting a vocational dimension to the argument, while on the other hand the recommendations that better financial support may improve retention infers a more pragmatic view of the job market. The role of Nightingale in shaping modern nursing was less explicit than at the time of writing the first book, and new nursing role models were apparent in recruitment drives such as of Claire Bertschinger, a highly acclaimed nurse who worked for the International Red Cross at the frontline of famine relief in Ethiopia, where she made heartbreaking choices but inspired a generation with her courage. Indeed she encapsulated the unspoken spirit of both Nightingale and Seacole's work in the Crimea. Twenty modern nursing champions named by the Nursing Times in 2008 included a mix of influential policy makers, educators, practitioners, activists and academics. The profile of white women was still maintained with three men and one black woman bucking the trend (Nursing Times 2008).

Nightingale's role in the shaping of modern nursing was deemed sufficiently important and influential to merit a detailed discussion in Chapter 1. Quoting Abel-Smith (1960) I described her role as a response to the need to create a respectable profession for a surplus of upper middle-class women in the mid-nineteenth century. Nursing became that respectable profession but from early on was dominated by a class hierarchy and later 'racial insignia' (in the sense of race being seen as a visible badge of difference alongside class and gender) reflected in nurses' positions and locations (Carpenter 1977).

It was not until the post–Second World War era that 'racial insignia' began to play an explicit role in the creation of nursing divisions and disadvantage. An enduring model of nurse training was developed in the élite voluntary hospitals to train matrons as leaders of bedside nurses. In Carpenter's view this model came about because care work was regarded as lower class but 'carried out under the moral leadership of upper class women' (Carpenter 1977, p. 168). During the 1980s, there was a huge drop in nurses training in the UK as part of general government disinvestment in the NHS. This drop coincided with the demographic time bomb and the decline of the traditional pool of eighteen–year-old female recruits, the phasing out of apprentice-style training and the introduction of Project 2000.

Active recruitment of overseas nurses was one of the key strategies to meet ambitious targets set out by 'New Labour' in their NHS Plan for 2000 to increase the workforce.[10] In the seven years to March 2005 over 71,000 nurses educated outside the UK registered with the Nursing and Midwifery Council, which represented 37% of all new registrants (NMC 2005a). Total new registrations climbed fast from 1998/9, and most of the increase was initially constituted by registrations of nurses educated outside the EU. By 2005, although overseas registrations had fallen slightly, they remained high at over 11,000 per annum (NMC 2005a). In the intervening years till the time of writing, there has been a gradual slow down in international recruitment, with the government in 2006 no longer designating nursing as a 'shortage' profession.

The experiences of migrant nurses, who had come to the UK as part of this active recruitment drive, can be used as a lens to comment on the globalization of the workforce, the current state of UK nursing and the interface between nursing and caring (Allan and Larsen 2003, Smith et al. 2006, Smith and Mackintosh 2007). These findings shed light on whether modern nursing continues to be in Nightingale's image or under her shadow. Allan (2007) suggests that in an increasingly competitive global labour market, when faced with a nursing shortage the UK government supported the recruitment of overseas trained nurses as a consequence of a care gap which had arisen from several policy shifts during the 1990s and the inherent tension which exists in the UK rhetoric, which claims that caring is at the heart of nursing. Rather Allan found that the 'ideal type' of British nursing had been shaped historically by a discourse of caring associated with Nightingale, which located the essence of nursing very firmly in the bedside delivery of nursing care and was particularly common among overseas nurses who had trained in the former colonial countries of Africa and Australasia. This discourse of caring has resonances with contradictions described previously by Carpenter (1977) that care work was seen as 'a lower class activity' led by 'the upper class'. Filipina nurses offer a particularly interesting contradiction since they were portrayed as caring and gentle and 'excellent bedside nurses', but in reality their United States-style education equips them with highly developed technical skills which get obscured by gender and racial stereotyping (Choy 2003, Smith et al. 2006, Allan et al. 2009).

Summary

In this chapter I have described the sort of people who trained as nurses at City Hospital in the 1980s and how their gender, class and ethnic characteristics are associated with the history of the institution in which they worked. I have updated these data from a number of studies and databases[11] to show that the recent workforce profile has changed (Smith et al. 2006). The gender division remains roughly similar, but there is now a significant percentage of mature students (26 years and over) and a migrant workforce of overseas trained nurses who contribute their perspectives on caring and diversity of experiences to the students' learning environment.

I have also briefly described the methods I used to study the patients, students, nurses and teachers at the City Hospital and school of nursing and student nurse learning and clinical leadership in four universities.

Next I have shown ways in which the Nightingale image was perpetuated at City Hospital through the job prospectus, selection and assessment procedures. In the climate of the 2000s, although recruitment interviews are still an important aspect of selection, now a range of nursing recruits bring a varied background of academic qualifications and work experiences, including a significant number of recruits who have worked as HCAs prior to applying for nurse training. The motivation to care and experience of 'people work' are still seen to be important factors both by the people who apply to become nurses and by those who select them.

Examining patients' images of nurses showed in the first study how they colluded in the perpetuation of the image of the nurse as having 'natural' skills and being vocationally motivated and dedicated 'natural' carers. Students vigorously rejected the view that they were vocationally motivated to become nurses. Now the discourse is dominated by nursing's entry into higher education, where it is subject to academic scrutiny, professional regulation particularly in relation to assessment and mentorship and a public discourse that has suggested that nurses may have become 'too posh to wash'.

How then are the gender, occupational and caring ideologies, past and present, reflected in the current students' plan of training? And can they still learn to care?

Nothing is really said about care: defining nursing knowledge

The title for this chapter was derived from data in the first study in which I found that the students who were recruited to City Hospital came with a commitment to care but also to be students in an 'academically demanding' environment. Since then a number of major changes have transformed nursing knowledge and practice, and the teaching and learning process. These changes include the introduction of two new curricula which involved a move from apprenticeship training in the National Health Service (NHS) to university-based education and supernumerary student status. During this transition the Nursing and Midwifery Council (NMC) has played a major role in defining the structure and content of the curriculum through standard setting and regulation and has shifted the emphasis from biomedical knowledge to encompass people-orientated knowledge. Workforce issues persist in which the students are caught between the competing demands of learning and caring and the two different worlds of the school and the ward that have given way to an alternative discourse that describes an 'uncoupling' of higher education from the clinical sector (Allan et al. 2008a).

The chapter reviews the structure and content of nurse education at two different periods, traces the influences that have shaped the nursing curricula and describes how students and their teachers perceive the many changes in policy and practice. Students in the 1980s did not expect that they would so quickly and so soon be counted in the workforce for more than 80 per cent of their training. They were full-time classroom students for only 30 out of 156 weeks and a sixth of that was right at the beginning of training in the Foundation Unit. The rest of the time was spent in the wards giving patient care, where they made up two-thirds of the workforce. The experience of finding themselves as principal care givers provoked two reactions. One was that they, the student nurses, were the group of people who cared the most since there were more of them. Second, they resented that their learning role was secondary to their role as workers. One student told me angrily, 'You go on the ward. You're not the student nurse at all. You're the workforce and if you learn something then good for you'.

A tutor also observed:

> Student nurses don't want to be used as pairs of hands but to have their learning role recognized, that's the problem, and here at City we depend on them as the workforce.

The impact of policy on nurse education and the nursing workforce

When the first study took place, the school of nursing – the teaching arm of nurse education – and the clinical areas – the practice arm of student learning – were geographically, ideologically and administratively close and both part of the National Health Service (NHS). Since the introduction of Project 2000 in the 1990s, this is no longer the case. Schools of nursing are now based in the universities while the NHS continues to provide the majority of the clinical placements in which students ostensibly play a supernumerary rather than a direct workforce role but where their labour rather than their learning often takes precedence. Indeed, some students reported feeling split loyalties as to whether they identified with the university or with the NHS through their NHS 'Home' trust where they were allocated for their clinical practice. The students' feelings of split loyalties are hardly surprising given their designated supernumerary status and the 50:50 split between the theory-based curriculum and work-based learning. The students were not the only ones who felt a 'split' between education and practice. Their nursing lecturers reported both a lack of clinical engagement and only occasional contact with students during placements because of a combination of university commitments and a programme structure which accentuated the separation between theory and practical experience and the 'uncoupling' of higher education from the clinical sector (Allan et al. 2008a).

One of the educational leaders was concerned that these spilt loyalties were confusing for both students and staff and were compounded by the requirement to spend 2,300 hours over three years in clinical practice thereby effectively, in her view, providing 'free labour' and making them 'feel they belong to the hospital'.

If the service staff viewed the students as 'free labour' then it is hardly surprising that they constantly felt the need to negotiate and re-negotiate their supernumerary status. Survey findings revealed that many students perceived supernumerary status to be a theoretical entitlement that was often absent in practice, and they felt used as a 'spare pair of hands'.

Trained nurses were described as 'too busy to teach with no time to explain some procedures'. But when the staffing levels were good, students were able 'to enjoy any and all learning opportunities as they arose'.

Caring not nursing, working not learning

The change in the division of labour since the first study took place and the introduction of health care assistants (HCA) into the nursing workforce meant that students experienced role confusion on some shifts. If, for example, there were staff nurses and students on the shift and no HCAs and many highly dependent patients then the student would be expected to take on the HCA role. Other times when there was a shortage of qualified staff students found themselves being asked to 'make up the numbers of Registered Nurses (RN) and left to carry out the role of the RN which makes it very difficult and causes anxiety'.

A third year student reported that when there was 'a lack of qualified staff and low staffing levels...I was never supernumerary because I was used to make up the numbers which meant I missed some learning opportunities because I was too busy to leave the ward'.

Supernumerary status is defined by the NMC as the expectation by pre-registration students to work with mentors who are required to supervise them at all times, either directly or indirectly (NMC 2004c, NMC 2008a, 2010c). This definition clearly leads to confusion as to whether the student is part of the workforce or a supernumerary student whose principal task is to learn.

In the current study, supernumerary status was not viewed by most qualified staff as a legitimate way of being a student nurse; rather they felt that students should be learning to give direct nursing care to patients in the same way they had learnt as student nurses and to be ready to work immediately on registration as fully competent practitioners. Students aspiring to supernumerary status as stated in their formal curriculum found themselves being expected to give hands-on care, often with minimum supervision and mentor support. Supernumerary status was highlighted by staff as problematic because they perceived it as impeding students' acquisition of clinical competencies, compounded by their attitudes to care delivery which they said students saw as conflicting with their learning role. They also said that students gave them mixed messages: on the one hand some students reported they were being given too much responsibility while on the other there were those who considered their 'hands on' experience to be insufficient. Many students described themselves as wanting to care and willing to learn, but they were clear they were able to do so only if the trained staff, and in particular their mentors supported them in their learning endeavours. There was yet another group of students, described in Chapter 5, which recognized the competing demands on the qualified staff to administer the technical

and administrative tasks in an increasi
the same time assisting students to lear
their future role as registered nurses. T
selves to protect their mentors by not pu
support them when the shift was busy.

Sharples (2009) suggests that the rea
numerary status is the automatic assump
the workforce equates with not participa
NMC, student status means that:

> Students undertaking programmes of prep
> out by the approved educational instituti
> practice settings to enable them to achiev... ...ne required standards of proficiency.
> Supernumerary status means that the student shall not as part of their programme of
> preparation be employed by any person or body under a contract of service to provide
> nursing care (NMC 2004c, p. 19).

Supernumerary status therefore means students are no longer employed as paid
members of the workforce as in the past but nor does it prevent them from fully
participating in providing hands-on nursing as a part of learning through doing.
The NMC also specifies that.

> Experiences should be educationally led and the supernumerary status of students
> maintained. Registrants acting as mentors are responsible for ensuring that public
> protection is paramount and are accountable for their decisions to delegate work to
> students. In addition to mentors students are also required to have personal tutors to
> support their learning in both academic and practice environments and be involved in
> assessing their standards of proficiency to enter the register.

Thus the NMC clearly distinguishes between two different learning environments – academic and practice – which correspond to the two different worlds of
school and ward.

In the first study the 'different worlds' of school and ward were particularly
apparent in which the nurse teachers inhabited the airy classrooms and quiet
corridors of the school and were rarely seen in the hustle and bustle of the
wards. Students frequently referred to the wards as 'out there' – which symbolized the 'real' world of patients and nurses, doctors and diseases. Sitting in the
hushed silence of the comfortable school library surrounded by books, the wards
did indeed seem a world away rather than the five-minute walk to the adjacent
building.

Often when I walked between the hospital and the school in 'off research'
times, I would meet nurses hurrying either on or off duty. They would often stop
to fill me in with the most recent events that I had 'missed' on the ward. Had

had another respiratory arrest? Wasn't it terrible that Mr
nly deteriorated in the night and died? Or the news that Lisa
sment, but Mary got a terrible report and is really upset. Then I
t the school minutes later in order to check the timetable to select
s I was going to observe. Titles like 'Passing a Naso-Gastric Tube',
ysiology of the Blood' or 'How to nurse patients with this or that disease'
quently appeared. Sessions that might have dealt with the feelings around a
udden death, a respiratory emergency or a failed assessment were less easy to
identify. Was this why students complained that 'school's got nothing to do with
nursing' or that their teachers did not have enough to do with them on the wards,
leading them to conclude that 'It's two different worlds'?

The separateness and difference between the two worlds of school and ward
has become even more polarized by the ideological and geographical distance
evident in the second study. In all four study sites, the universities were located
some miles and an hour's journey away from the clinical areas where we undertook our mini-ethnographies and interviewed the lecturers. In the post-Project
2000 era, difference was emphasized by distance between universities and clinical areas but also because they were no longer part of the same organization as
they had been in the past.

While undertaking fieldwork it was possible to get a sense of students and
staff coming on and off duty while walking the hospital corridors to and from the
wards, but one week was too short a period to get to know them in the way that I
had been able to engage with participants during my study of City Hospital. It was
also possible to get a sense of a clinical teaching presence through the Practice
Educators (PE) whose explicit role was to facilitate student learning during their
placements and maintain links with the university. The PEs were NHS employees which in itself served to emphasize the distinction between educational and
clinical institutions. Their office was based in the hospital, and they readily provided me with a desk, internet and telephone access during the fieldwork. The
PEs spent the majority of their time in the wards, visiting students and organizing
tutorials and seminars, and it was evident that they provided the main contact for
the students and staff.

Contemporary students saw practice and the university as two separate entities
with their supernumerary status, allowing them to distinguish between learning
and working. They also differentiated between university and practice learning.
One such example was from a student who commented that she learnt more from
her clinical placement in a hospice than she did 'at university'. Over the years,
researchers have explained why students experience dissonance between the two
learning environments in the way the student describes. Eraut (1985) suggested
it was because there had been a lack of understanding that the formal knowledge
acquired in the classroom was different from the informal knowledge acquired in
practice. More recently Evans and colleagues (2009) found that formal knowledge

could be successfully re-contextualized
a teacher to assist in its translation and

The current study shows that there a
staff to come and go easily between the
ing that the opportunities for the re-cont
ited. The PE, however, provided a visit
During fieldwork there was little sense of
despite the stated role of the link lectur
and practice. When students were asked f
ment experiences, the link lecturer was id
throughout the placement. It's easy to feel
the link between theory and practice' and
ants understand what "supernumerary" means'.

The link lecturers for their part said that financial, administrative and legal
factors shaped the way they interpreted their roles.

One link lecturer said her role was to 'support students in practice, support
mentors and audit ward environments, not to work with students or to be practice
role models. In the current financial circumstances we've been advised to lessen
our actual presence on the wards'.

Another nurse teacher who described herself as 'feeling caught' between the
different aspirations, requirements, time pressures and financial systems of the
university and the service said:

> It wasn't long ago we were expected to go and do so many clinical hours a year to
> keep up our competence. But then the question began to be asked 'how can we as a
> university afford to do that? So that's what stopped it; and it was just getting harder
> and harder to find the time to fit it all in.

Because of a lack of understanding of the link lecturer's role in practice, it had
been left up to individual teachers to resolve differing expectations and conflicts
with their clinical colleagues. As one lecturer put it:

> I think you have to be careful to explain to people that there are many legal reasons
> why you can't just give patient care; I'm not a trust employee, I can't just walk in there.
> So it is important to understand that the link lecturer role is not the clinical teacher
> role. But I think there's a yearning for that role when the clinical teacher used to come
> and work with the students so as to take the pressure off the staff.

Although the students in both studies had minimal contact with the school
and their teachers during their clinical placements, the difference was that in
the 1980s they continued to experience their influence at an ideological level
throughout training. The school set the 'ideals and standards' of the City nurse
and designed the formal content of their training to achieve them. There was not

mpeting pressures from a variety of educational, service
ganizations each with their own systems of governance and
ating anxiety, uncertainty and conflicting expectations as there
00s.

teacher in the 1980s could 'just walk in' to the ward at any time.
al teachers, although school based, were employed to work with the stu-
ts in practice. This role has long since been disbanded, but as the link lecturer says it is a role that is still yearned for.

As described in Chapter 1, national nursing ideologies in the 1980s rejected
the image of the nurse as the doctor's assistant based on the medical treatment of
disease, in favour of the 'new' nurse committed to care and interpersonal relationships with patients. An alternative knowledge base for nursing was sought which
turned away from a biomedical one.[1]

In the immediate period following the completion of the first study, a number
of approaches to the curriculum emerged based on three influential documents.
The first was the Project 2000: A New Preparation for Practice (UKCC 1986),
a document underpinned by a philosophy of health and the need for students to
become supernumerary 'knowledgeable doers'. Other approaches were based on
the recommendations of the Making a Difference (Department of Health 1999)
and Fitness for Practice (UKCC 1999) documents with their focus on clinical
competences and tasks and mechanisms for supervising students in practice.
Fitness for Practice was the outcome of the UKCC review of pre-registration nursing programmes and a more sympathetic interpretation of the 'Too posh to wash'
lobby described in Chapter 2, in that it highlighted the lack of confidence experienced by students on newly qualifying and suggested this was because their
education, particularly during practice, had not been organized adequately to
support and prepare them for the demands and pressures of modern health care.

As the recent fieldwork progressed it became apparent that the setting of
'ideals and standards' for student nurse learning in the 2000s were done not
by individual schools of nursing but the NMC via the university lecturers and
implemented in practice by the PEs and mentors, as the 'de facto' guardians of
the NMC standards and protectors of the public. The mentors were required to
ensure the students achieved the levels of competence specified as learning outcomes to become safe practitioners.

So my impression was that nursing ideology in the 2000s was characterized
as policy and target driven, and it was less easy to identify the underlying nursing ideologies, philosophies and knowledge base underpinning the curriculum
in a society that had become highly regulated, workforce driven and competence
based. In an NMC Mapping Paper (2005b) a number of these frameworks and
benchmarks were identified as key to the pre-registration nursing curriculum
and mapped against the NMC Standards of Proficiency. These were the QAA
Subject Benchmark Statements for Healthcare Programmes and two Department

of Health Frameworks: Knowledge and Skills (KSF) and Ten Essential Shared Capabilities for the Mental Health Workforce. I was left with the impression that nursing in the 2000s finds itself squeezed between higher education and professional regulation, and the potentially competing demands of government, education and the profession. What then are the effects on curriculum development and the content of nurse education?

As Sharples (2009) observes, the NMC decides on the core content and outcomes of the pre-registration nursing curriculum, and the overall structure of the programme for all universities. The main recommendations from the *Fitness for Practice* (UKCC 1999) report have been revised over the years, although many of the key principles still feature within current programme guidelines based on two key documents. The first is the NMC *Standards of Proficiency for Pre-registration Nursing Education* (NMC 2004c, 2009), 'the gold standard' for how nurses are trained and the criteria on which programme quality is controlled and monitored. The standards are also said to be 'underpinned by guiding principles that establish the philosophy and values of the NMC's requirements for programmes leading to registration as a nurse' (2004c, p. 13). These principles include the primacy of practice, theory and practice integration, evidence-based practice and learning, provision and management of care, a 'health for all' orientation and a lifelong learning approach.

The second element in the NMC orientation is the *Essential Skills Clusters for Pre-registration Nursing Programmes* (NMC 2007) of which there are five domains:

- Care, Compassion and Communication
- Organisational Aspects of Care
- Infection Prevention and Control
- Nutrition and Fluid Management
- Medicines Management

These *Essential Skills Clusters* (NMC 2007) lay down the standards or competency levels that are expected of students at two specific points in their nursing programme: first at the point of transfer from the Common Foundation Programme (CFP) to one of the four specialist branches in adult, mental health, children's or learning disability nursing, and second at the end of their branch programme when they complete their training and proceed to registration (NMC 2007).

Educators, whether involved in strategy, or teaching in the academic or practice setting were aware of the profound changes that had taken place in nurse education over the past decade (Allan et al. 2008a). A PE identified the prominent role played by government policy in the teaching of nursing ideology and how its implementation in practice had had a direct impact on the 'grassroots'.

For a nurse lecturer interviewed about patient safety, the overarching aim of nurse education was driven by the NMC's professional code of conduct and this meant:

> Right from the very beginning I teach about professional standards and professionalism and clinical governance, it's all in there because it has to be, because it's driven by our professional code (nurse lecturer quoted in Pearson et al. 2009).

The 'professional code' titled 'Standards of Conduct performance and ethics' has five statements outlining the NMC's expectations for all nurses (NMC 2008b). 'The Care of People' is seen as a priority, and nurses and midwives are expected to engender trust, maintain integrity and honesty, protect and promote health, 'provide a high standard of practice and care at all times' and 'uphold the reputation of your profession'. The emotional labour required to meet the NMC's expectations is inherent in the language and sentiment of the Code and in particular has resonances with Bolton's (2000) notion of 'prescriptive' emotion management as specified by organizations and professional rules of conduct described in Chapter 1.

In one nurse leader's opinion there was no longer a distinct knowledge base or discipline-specific subjects within the nursing curriculum that could be easily identified but rather an emphasis on educational delivery and how the students were taught and learnt:

> [Currently] there is a melding of subject matter; everything is integrated i.e. it is difficult to pick out the specific subjects they are taught but rather there is an emphasis on the way they are taught say through case studies or enquiry based learning.

As a reminder of the structure and content of nurse education in the 1980s, I return to my content analysis of nurse training in the original study followed by an analysis of how the contemporary curriculum is organized and delivered.

The content of nurse training

City Hospital in the 1980s

At the time of the first study, despite national patient-centred ideologies, the theoretical and practical organization of the three-year nursing programme at City was based on medical specialities, such as paediatrics, obstetrics, geriatrics, gynaecology and psychiatry, with the heaviest emphasis being given to four modules each of medical and surgical nursing in the first and final year of training. This in part explained why disease-orientated sessions dominated the timetables.

In my initial study I was also curious to find out how national and local nursing ideologies were reflected in the curriculum papers given to students at the beginning of training. These papers stated the general course philosophy and the aims, objectives and content of each of the 15 modules (see: Companion website, Appendix C, Smith 1992).

I also wanted to find out whether these ideologies were visible in the classroom by studying the timetables further, observing selected teaching sessions and interviewing teachers and students.

The curriculum papers reflected a dual picture of the new 'people-orientated' and the old 'biological' approaches to nursing. The modular aims and objectives demonstrated a commitment to meeting patients' physical, psychological and social needs, but the suggested content was dominated by the 'natural sciences' in the Foundation Unit and by the signs and symptoms, techniques and procedures associated with medical diagnosis and disease in the subsequent three-year programme.

They were more likely to describe nursing in terms of the 'basics', i.e. bed-making, bathing, mouth-care, lifting, feeding, toileting, *talking* and *empathy* with patients. One student proclaimed: 'Nursing isn't a dry boring subject ... we are talking about people'. Another student who believed that 'if people don't matter then you can't do nursing' described care as an essential part of nursing knowledge but was disappointed by its lack of conceptualization in the curriculum. She said, 'Nothing is really said about care. They [the tutors] say you have to care but nobody actually says what caring is'.

At this early stage of training students still clearly related to the selection criteria that had played an important part in their recruitment to train at City Hospital, i.e. their interest in and experience of working with people.

After six months of training, students talked about knowing 'the basics by now' and needing to know about different techniques and investigations. The knowledge required to nurse was described as 'the solid facts, the diseases, the anatomy and the physiology'.

The students' comments were indicative of a shift in emphasis during the first year away from so-called basics and people work to the 'solid facts' of 'theory' and the techniques and procedures of practice. One student in her third year used Advanced Level biology as a yardstick by which to measure the knowledge and 'absolute facts' that she believed were being 'missed out' in her training programme. She said, 'I did biology up to A level so I do know how much I should know ... I want higher knowledge from the school ... somewhere the absolute facts are being missed out'.

Two other third-year students expressed similar doubts about the state of their knowledge, because they judged it on the basis of its medical and technical content. One of them concluded:

Although you spend a lot of time building up your nursing skills, the depth of knowledge into diseases, drugs and therapy gets rather left by the wayside and I find that my knowledge is really sort of patchy and scanty and there is no sort of depth to it. I've just learnt bits here and there.

This student identified her time on the ward as the place where she built up her nursing skills through practical experience. But she saw these skills as distinct from her 'patchy and scanty' knowledge base which she judged on a biomedical model of 'disease, drugs and therapy'.

Why then did students shift to judging nursing on the basis of biomedical rather than people-orientated knowledge? One explanation seemed to lie in the way in which their nursing programme was designed around modules based on medical specialities and a curriculum dominated by biomedical knowledge.

The NHS in the 2000s

How then did the content and structure of the curriculum differ in the 2000s? What does the current curriculum content tell us about current nursing ideologies and philosophies? The discussion so far suggests that the NMC has the power and influence to prescribe what nurses do through the content and structure of the pre-registration curriculum by laying down standards of proficiency against levels of essential skills to be achieved and a code of conduct which goes beyond individual institutions (NMC 2004c, 2008b). In terms of the curriculum the NMC (2004c, p. 19) states that in order to provide a knowledge base for practice a number of contemporary theoretical perspectives need to be explored such as:

- professional, ethical and legal issues
- the theory and practice of nursing
- the context in which health and social care is delivered
- organizational structures and processes
- communication
- social and life sciences relevant to nursing practice
- frameworks for social care provision and care systems

Further elaboration of these perspectives makes it quite clear that there is no choice in the matter and that the content of the curriculum has to reflect contemporary knowledge and enable development of evidence-based practice though strategies for integrating knowledge and skills gained in both academic and practice environments. Nursing education therefore *must guarantee* that the person (i.e. the nurse) has acquired:

- adequate knowledge of the sciences on which general nursing is based, including sufficient understanding of the structure, physiological functions and behaviour of healthy and sick persons, and of the relationship between the state of health and physical and social environment of the human being;

- sufficient knowledge of the nature and ethics of the profession and of general principles of health and nursing;
- adequate clinical experience, such experience which should be selected for its training value, should be gained under the supervision of qualified nursing staff and in places where the number of qualified staff and equipment are appropriate for the nursing care of the patients;
- the ability to participate in the practical training of health personnel and experience of working with such personnel and
- the experience of working with members of other professions in the health sector.

How then are these perspectives and specifications applied in practice? In order to get a sense of the curriculum changes in the intervening years a content analysis of online curriculum documents was undertaken, mentoring training documents and QAA reports since the introduction of Project 2000 and the Fitness for Practice curricula for the four case studies. In the new electronic age, the content and structure of the curricula and how students are assessed are available on university websites which give an indication of the public face of nursing.

The curriculum in four case study sites

During the curriculum analysis trends were identified which clearly reflected the NMC perspectives and specifications (NMC 2004c). Each of the programmes were offered at degree or diploma level, were three years in length, divided between 50 per cent theory and 50 per cent practice (a minimum of 4,600 hours total) and validated by the NMC. The entry qualifications for degree programmes were typically three 'A' levels at grade B or C or equivalent. Access to diploma programmes was possible through National Vocational Qualifications and Foundation degrees as part of the widening participation agenda, a route popular with former HCAs.

Although the detail of the programmes varied between the four sites, the overall structure was the same. The first year consisted of a common foundation, followed by a two-year specialist branch in adult, mental health or children's nursing. Each programme had a modular structure with core competences and outcomes based on the NMC's (2004c) requirements for registration – i.e. knowledge, understanding and skills with specific reference to clinical competence, high standards of nursing care, working in multidisciplinary teams and attainment of professional attributes with an overall emphasis of producing a safe practitioner.

In terms of the programme content, biological science was no longer seen as the predominant knowledge base of nursing, but there was now a requirement to balance it with psychology and sociology as part of the 'scientific basis of nursing'. The documents also specified the acquisition of a range of research, communication and clinical skills, in diverse placement settings (acute and community) and patient conditions across the life cycle. The importance of evidence-based practice was also mentioned in all documents in addition to the importance of integrating theory and practice.

The following types of learning described in the curriculum documents were in line with the stakeholder's view above that method might appear to 'meld' or overshadow content. Types of learning included lifelong adult collaborative action learning, problem-based, enquiry-based and reflective learning, as well as the use of direct clinical and indirect practical experience to link theory and practice. Learning and teaching strategies included traditional lectures and seminars and a range of interactive strategies such as scenarios for enquiry-based learning seminars, learning contracts, reflective diaries and portfolios, computer-assisted learning, e-learning and the practice of skills through simulation, role play and presentations in clinical skills labs. During their placements, students were allocated a designated mentor who had completed a course of training recognized by the NMC to facilitate their work-based learning (NMC 2010c).

In terms of programme structure the following themes were identified: linking theory and practice; mentoring systems and training; supernumerary status and student support. We elaborate each theme below.

Linking theory and practice

With the Fitness for Practice curriculum came a different ratio of theory to practice. The previous 60:40 ratio in favour of theory in the Project 2000 curriculum had been modified to 50:50. The learning that takes place in practice was given due credit through this change, and each university used student portfolios to link theory and practice learning. One university stated that the portfolio provided 'a record of significant learning experiences' and 'provides the basis for discussion with the student's mentor'. Another university stated that 'the student portfolio was designed and developed to assist students to gain optimal learning in practice' as well as 'to provide evidence of learning'. The content of the student's portfolio included the nine core skills of clinical practice prescribed by the NMC and clustered into 'Nine Practice Skills Areas'. The selection of these nine areas had been influenced by the Department of Health's Essence of Care publication on clinical governance (Department of Health 2001, NHS Modernisation Agency 2003) defined as:

1. Principles of self care
2. Personal and oral hygiene
3. Food and nutrition
4. Continence and bladder and bowel care
5. Pressure ulcers
6. Safety of clients/patients with mental health needs
7. Record keeping
8. Privacy and dignity
9. Communication

The Essence of Care, launched in February 2001, was part of the NHS Plan and provided a toolkit to help practitioners to take a structured approach through patient-focused benchmarking to share and compare practice. The idea of the toolkit was to enable practitioners to identify best practice and to develop action plans where there were areas for improvement. Patients and professionals worked together to agree on what they considered best practice in the **softer aspects of care,** which were deemed crucial to ensuring patients had a quality experience and that **the basics of care** were achieved (my emphases: communication and the emotional components of professional care are being designated as 'softer' and linked to the 'basics').

The aim of the Essence of Care Toolkit was to provide a mechanism to recognize and spread best practice, across the NHS as part of its commitment to *drive up quality* (again my emphasis: the connection between quality and care is being made). The nine areas addressed by The Essence of Care are seen as fundamental to achieving the basics of care necessary for quality improvement and integral to clinical governance.

The portfolio also presented the KSF Framework (Department of Health 2004b, p. 8) with its six dimensions designated as core essential skills and listed as:

1. Communication
2. Personal and people development
3. Health safety and security
4. Service Development
5. Quality
6. Equality, diversity and rights

As already noted, the mentors may be regarded as the 'de facto' guardians of these NMC standards and protectors of the public by ensuring the students achieve the levels of competence specified.

Mentoring systems and training

To ensure the students achieve the prescribed levels of confidence, they must be allocated a designated mentor during placements to facilitate their work-based learning (NMC 2010c). In line with this orientation each university curriculum document identified the mentor as the key to practice learning. For example, in terms of locating responsibility for student success, one university reiterated the Making a Difference document's (Department of Health 1999) position that 'the mentor is the arbiter of the students' success or otherwise in practice'. The NMC views the mentor as playing a critical role in protecting the students' supernumerary status, rendering them free from employment obligations of the past and the direct control of their labour by the ward sister.

Supernumerary status

Although the students' need for supernumerary status was prescribed in the curriculum documents, there appeared to be an underlying tension or ambivalence between what the universities' saw on the one hand was the need to learn and on the other as the requirement to work. This tension reflects the confusion surrounding supernumerary status as described earlier in this chapter. Each university's documentation gave clear guidelines as to the definition of supernumerary status. One university document stated that it did 'not include the students being counted in the number of nurses required to deliver the service; the Trust does not pay for the student to work; the student's educational needs are considered paramount and take precedence over service needs'. However the student was reminded that 'it is important to understand that you [the student] are not an onlooker. The experience of giving care as a helpful participant, and being part of a team of health professionals is vital to your learning'. This phrase is most telling, given the tensions and ambiguities surrounding supernumerary status revealed in both interview and questionnaire findings. And yet it seems that in at least this one university the concept of supernumerary status was found to be troubling and difficult to balance. On the one hand there was a firm statement that the student was a learner and on the other a suggestion that learning as part of a team while delivering care was vital to learning. The recognition that students should be supported during this process was articulated in a variety of ways in all four documents.

Student support

The range of student support interventions included a continuum of pastoral support by personal tutors through to university-wide student support agencies.

However there were some differences in the emphasis that each university placed on the type of support offered. For example, one university stated that in placements mentors were the first line of support followed by clinical placement facilitators and clinical placement development managers. The ward manager was not described as having a role. In contrast, another university's first statement about student support stated that the personal tutor was the main student support alongside the academic support available from the Dyslexia Support Unit and Student Advice Centre. The guidance in another university document mentioned the mentor as the main source of student support and a fourth mentioned that 'practical skills will be taught by nurses working in the area of placement along with lecturers from the College who have a formal link with the placements'. This was the only reference to the link lecturer role in all four documents.

It is clear from analyzing these documents that the universities demonstrated the tensions and ambiguities associated with linking theory and practice, mentoring systems and training, supernumerary status and student support. Some of the universities attempted to address the student's position caught between practice and academe through the provision of on-line learning opportunities, access to on-line communities of practice and guidance on the student role which gave a sense of 'support at a distance'.

Implementing the 'Living Curriculum'

The 1980s

In the original study I undertook an analysis of the timetables planned by the nurse tutors as one way of assessing how the written curriculum also became a reality in the classroom. The analysis showed that the content of their teaching sessions, with the exception of some of the specialities, such as psychiatry, during the second year, closely corresponded with the biomedically orientated curriculum.

During the Foundation Unit and medical modules for example, I found that only 14 per cent of all sessions could be categorized as dealing with a more people-orientated approach to care (see: Companion website, Appendix D, Smith 1992). The content of these sessions emphasized such topics as the principles and practice of the nursing process, interpersonal communication, experiential learning, nursing care of patients in pain and the management of death and dying. I assumed that during these sessions students learnt about the conceptualization of nursing as care and 'people' work. I chose to observe some of these sessions in order to test my assumption.

Nursing process: philosophy, conceptual device or work method?

First of all, I wanted to find out to what extent the nursing process philosophy and work method was used as a device for conceptualizing nursing knowledge and practice as care and 'people' work by both teachers and their students. The evidence provided by the timetables (1% of all sessions) suggested hardly at all. There were very few sessions which fitted in with the underlying conceptual framework of the nursing process such as Henderson's (1960) and Roper's (1976) models for nursing practice based on the activities of daily living.[2]

During interviews with tutors I began to understand why the nursing process did not feature prominently as an integral part of their teaching or as a way of conceptualizing nursing. Many of them interpreted it in different ways. One tutor described the nursing process as about 'feelings and attitudes and more applicable to the ward'.

Another tutor explained that nurse tutors were having difficulties with the nursing process because of insufficient preparation to use it either in the classroom or ward. Actually, she admitted,

'I do like the medical model and it can be nice and logical and it's scientific and you can do that in school beautifully. I don't think we can throw the medical model out completely because at the end of the day we've got people coming in to hospital with diseases. We've gone overboard thinking it's the person we must look at'.

This tutor's reaction was interesting because she, like many of her colleagues, was finding difficulty conceptualizing nursing as people-orientated knowledge. Her view that the medical model can be 'logical' and 'scientific' implied that the nursing process, as an alternative model for conceptualizing knowledge, was not.

The students, therefore, had very little reason to view the nursing process as part of the theoretical content of their training, even during the first six months when they clearly related to nursing as people work. To them it was 'a waffly subject that all boils down to common sense in the end' or 'what you do really'. Even though the nursing process offered the potential for identifying and generating people-orientated knowledge, the students did not see it used in this way by their tutors. They began to regard it as 'common sense' and 'what you do' rather than an approach to nursing with its own knowledge base and set of skills.

The 2000s

In the recent study there was occasional reference by the students to Roper's model of nursing and the Activities of Daily Living, but they were not strong themes. The Nursing Process did not feature as either a philosophy or work method. The specification of standards of proficiency and essential skills clusters which consistently included communication, compassion, care and prioritization of patient need as essential nursing competences in the benchmarks, frameworks and code of conduct set out by statutory and government bodies were such that there was no option for them but to be included in the curriculum as the 'gold standard' of how nurses are trained and the quality of their curriculum is controlled and monitored (Sharples 2009). However these competence frameworks did not provide the same opportunity as the nursing process, activities of daily living and Roper's nursing model as a means of conceptualizing nursing. They were however what had potentially taken their place.

Affective/psychosocial nursing and learning to do emotional labour

In the first study I categorized the sessions on the timetables which dealt with affective/psychosocial nursing (10% of the total), and I assumed that students were likely to learn about the conceptualization of nursing as care and people work. I chose to observe some of these sessions in order to find out whether these were so, and to see how they related to the notion of training students to do emotional labour. I present extracts from two of these sessions below.

Patient–nurse perceptions: first-year students

This session was led by a tutor who was a psychiatric nurse specialist. She had specifically been asked to do this session by the general nurse teachers because they believed the topic required psychiatric expertise. Perception was defined at the beginning of the session as 'the interpretations and judgments made by nurses through observation of the way patients behave'.

> S(tudent). Patients don't know how to react to you when you go on to ward wearing your own clothes on your day off.
> T(utor). Why do you think that is?
> S. Well, what you wear is associated with your role; like wearing my uniform is associated with my role as a nurse.

The tutor agrees, then, reflecting on the nurse's role, asks:

Does X [refers to a senior teacher by name] still have that thing that you should smile the whole time?

S.   Yes she still has it.

T.   No wonder patients are confused! [She laughs.]

Another student then considers the effects nurses have on patients and comments 'It's dangerous the authority nurses have over patients'.

When she is asked to explain what she means, she replies:

Some patients become 'pets'. We all do it. They're looked at as 'very nice'. Or other patients get the reputation of being awkward and then you think 'well sister should know her work. If that's her opinion I'd better avoid him'.

S.   Often you find it's not true what they [trained staff] tell you.

S.   We as beginners are very vulnerable and on the side of the patients. Staff nurses have seen it all before and think patients are up to their 'old tricks'.

The content of this extract is interesting in terms of its association with learning to do emotional labour. Nurses were cast in a role symbolized by their uniforms. Tutor and students were aware that one of the senior teachers expected them to smile. The importance of smiling as a key 'caring' behaviour was reminiscent of Hochschild's descriptions of emotional labour in the airline industry. Flight attendants were also encouraged to smile by their instructors.

Differences between the two groups of workers (nurses and flight attendants) became apparent, however, as the students described the 'authority' they felt they had over patients. The hierarchical relationships within the British health care system determined the feeling rules surrounding certain patients. At the beginning of training, students saw themselves as vulnerable and on the side of the patient. But patients could acquire either positive or negative labels which were often legitimized by the trained staff's view of them. Because the students felt that the ward sister 'should know her job' and the staff nurses had seen it all before, they as the juniors should take their cues from them. In the case of the 'awkward' patient they felt that in order to conform to the rules and reduce internal conflicts, they should withdraw their emotional labour by avoiding him.

These strategies were very different from the official ones taught to flight attendants. They also recognized and labelled difficult passengers, but were formally taught to manage anger or irritation through deep acting techniques to enable them to continue their interaction. As the next account illustrates, students at City were expected to learn experientially to induce or suppress feelings irrespective of how they felt about their relationships with patients or colleagues. The classroom sessions gave them the opportunity to describe their emotional work but gave them little knowledge or guidance on how to manage their feelings.

Critical incidents: third-year students

The use of critical incidents (Clamp 1980) as a teaching method was popular with the nurse teachers during the third year of training.[3] The purpose of the method was to encourage students in small group sessions, to draw on incidents from their ward work in order to learn about their feelings, behaviour and attitudes.

One tutor described the method in the following way:

If you control the discussion firmly enough without being seen to control it then you can pick out the things that you actually ought to draw attention to, the things that can be learnt from. The students have a variety and richness of experience to offer.

During the session, students did describe a range of feelings while in contact with patients, feelings such as fear (because an aggressive patient on night duty threatened to throw his bed at them), failure (at being unable to cope personally with an offensive patient) or *guilt* at escorting an abusive, uncooperative patient home from hospital and persuading his desperate relatives to take him back. The students received both peer group support and empathy during the session, because many could identify similar emotionally demanding situations. But the way in which they expressed their feelings suggested that support in retrospect was too late: they had needed it at the time, when the labour of maintaining an outward appearance of calm and competence had cost them emotionally dear.

The story concerned a student who felt guilty for persuading relatives on the advice of doctors to accept a desperately disturbed patient home from an acute surgical ward in a bid to have him admitted to a psychiatric hospital.

Discussing the session with me in an interview later that day, another student gave a mixed reaction. She said:

S. I was amazed at that incident, where Belle took that bloke home. I was almost speechless, because anyone who's a student nurse can understand.

PS. What do you mean?

S. Belle was still screwed up about what she might have done to the emotional side of the sister of that patient and she brought it up in a lecture and she wasn't supported.

I asked why?

S. How could she be? It was a conversation. Belle thought that because she said it out loud she could be supported. It's not enough to say 'Well it's the medical and trained staff's problem because it was their decision to send him home. You're not guilty. Don't feel guilty'. How can you not feel guilty! She knew that she shouldn't have taken him home. She was the one who in the end had to convince that woman to take her brother into a home that was falling apart. She was the one who made the promises to the woman that her brother would soon be transferred to the psychiatric hospital. I just felt so much for her. I thought 'Where were you when you found out that man was still at home?' Were you standing at the phone, or sitting at report and staff nurse just passed it on to you as a bit of gossip and your heart sank because you knew you were the one who had promised his sister?

I knew that the student who had been involved in the incident appeared very distressed as she described what had happened, and it is likely that the tutor arranged to see her to talk about it after the session.

The student who had participated in the session concluded:

S.   And what was that student told when she left that ward? 'We have a lot to thank you for'. They should be doing more than thanking her. She will probably have that memory always.

This vivid account of the feelings generated in one student by the recounting of a critical incident showed the potential power of the method in offering students insights into emotional labour and the management of feelings on the wards. It also shows the need for systematic follow-up of some incidents by teachers and the need for careful contact with students and staff on the wards to be available to offer support closer to when such incidents occur.

The psychiatric nursing module

In the 1980s all student nurses undertook a psychiatric nursing module as part of their training which came at the end of the second year and was singled out as being of particular significance. If students wished to become a mental health nurse they were required to undertake a post-registration specialist training. In the current set up students chose to become a mental health nurse during their pre-registration training by opting for the mental health branch. In the NMC mapping document referred to above there is a Mental Health Framework that is used to look at the competences for this branch of nursing. These competences include partnership working, providing user centred care, challenging inequality, respecting diversity and making a difference as part of nursing care delivery and management (NMC 2004c).

In the first study the aims of the psychiatric module clearly articulated nursing as people work prioritizing patients' psychological and social needs and identifying student needs in terms of emotional support. One tutor thought that the module emphasized the students' personal development more than at any other time of their training. She said:

There is something about the whole atmosphere of the psychiatric hospital which seems particularly good for them. It's the fact that someone values them as a person.

Someone values their contribution, listens to what they say. It is so different from anything they've come across before. I think they get a lot of time and attention.

A student described the experience as teaching her 'a lot about the importance of talking to your patients and that sort of psychological side of their care. I think you are much more aware of it'.

The psychiatric module exposed students to an alternative knowledge base which was psychological and sociological in nature and translated into interpersonal and interviewing skills associated with people work. However, the module lasted only nine weeks, and unless the students returned to environments which valued the 'psychological side of care', they quickly readjusted to a biomedical view of nursing.[4]

Informal training for people work: feeling rules and emotion management

The psychiatric nursing module in the 1980s was too short to convince the majority of the students that they learnt their communication skills in any way other than informally. The most common examples given were those of role modelling and ward-based experience, and certainly not from classroom teaching or discussion.

First-year students told me:

You saw sister or staff nurse in some tricky situations with patients. They handled them so well. You *just* learnt by watching how they talked to them.

Or:

You see how the nurses sort of manage patients and talk to them and you *just* pick things up. It's *just* their general attitude; you think 'that's a really nice way to treat someone' ... and they show an example.

And again:

I think you just learn by watching the way other people do things, like talking to dying patients.

The point about all these comments is that the students might be seen to minimize the learning of emotional care by the repeated use of '*just* learning', '*just* picking it up', '*just* by watching', '*just* through experience'. An alternative explanation is that they apply the meaning of 'just' to these activities to infer the 'naturalness' of such learning as opposed to formal classroom teaching. The danger here is that the skills acquired through these activities might also be regarded as 'natural' and not requiring any or much skill to perform or effort to acquire.[5] A senior student said she also learnt by watching other people and identifying 'a good model'. She said:

> You think 'I'll remember that' or 'that's not the way I'd do it'. Then again it's almost inspirational or off the cuff.

The minimization of learning to respond to patients' emotional needs was also reflected in the belief that students brought with them the character and qualities to be able to care.

A first-year student at the time said:

> You have to be, even as a first warder, to have the character to be able to talk to strangers, and very quickly. If you haven't got that then I don't think you can nurse well.

> I think that if you're basically a caring person, which presumably you are if you come in to nursing, then I think you have your own sort of procedure. I don't think you should try and make everyone the 'standard' nurse.

Thus the students, just like their recruiters in Chapter 2, saw being a 'caring person' or 'able to talk to strangers' as part of the package that you brought with you as a nurse, not skills that had to be learnt and sustained. Teaching communication skills was seen by this last nurse, and by many of her colleagues, as taking away her personal communication style and replacing it with a 'standard' set of procedures.[6]

Two other students described expectations to be 'nice' to all patients. But they also recognized that there were circumstances under which they could not sustain one of the key characteristics of the City nurse, the capacity to remain 'on an even keel'.

The first-year student felt pressure to be 'nice' to patients. But she was quite clear that she would only be 'nice' to patients if as part of the equal exchange of 'niceness', they were also 'nice' to her. She said:

> I'll never say I particularly like all the patients. You're told you've got to be nice to them but I don't think you have to be if they're not being nice to you.

The student who had recently completed her training said:

> There are times when you're tired, you do and say things you wouldn't normally do. I remember the first time I snapped at a patient, I felt mortified, as I thought that nurses never show that they are personally hurt. Now I don't take that view.

The student identified 'when you're tired' as a time when she might 'do and say things' that weren't 'normal'. In other words she was describing conditions under which she could no longer induce or suppress her own feelings in deference to the patient's. She had found this a liberating experience in that she was able to acknowledge to herself that she had feelings that mattered. She also expressed a keen interest in people, their motivations and behaviours, and later went on to do a postgraduate qualification in psychiatric nursing.

The organization of mental health nursing is very different since the first study took place. Following the disbanding of the large psychiatric asylums, mental health nursing placements are predominantly based in the community and day care with only the acutely ill being hospitalized. During fieldwork I observed a second year 'mature' mental health nursing student's sensitive response to her adult branch colleague's 'stereotypical' view that 'teenage pregnancy' persisted because it was 'too easy' for young women who became pregnant to be helped with housing and receive generous state benefits. The mental health student was calm and quietly insistent that there was a need to understand that there might be a range of underlying emotional reasons why teenage women became pregnant. Her persistence and sensitivity was a living example of the NMC's expectations for 'mental health nurses to use a well developed and evidence-based repertoire of interpersonal, psychosocial and other skills that are underpinned by an empathetic attitude towards the service user' (NMC 2004c, p. 24).

Learning to communicate and emotion management: patients' views

Patients interviewed in the 1980s fell somewhere in between the view that nurses had to have certain qualities to be able to communicate with others, but also that part of their training should strengthen those qualities. A selection of comments that illustrate this point is presented below:

> The nurse has got to know her 'nursing' but the training must be right. Then it's her humanity immediately after that.
>
> You probably can't teach them to communicate, but you can advise them and if aspects of their personality will respond, you can teach them certain functions and give them hints and aids to guide them along those lines.
>
> It's got to be there [the ability to communicate] although I think you can mould it.

Thus the nurse had to have humanity, but her training had to be right, the type of personality that would respond to guidance, or an innate ability to communicate, which could then be moulded.

There were also those patients who gave a sense that the students were being trained to manage their emotions.

> You need to train nurses to care for people and not to panic.
>
> It's part of the training to learn to put up with a lot when dealing with old people. They can be cantankerous and the nurses need a lot of patience to hold it back.

Thus the nurse had to learn to care, but not to panic, and also to put up with a lot.

Patients' views: 2000

Patients interviewed for a patient safety study (Pearson et al., 2009) identified a variety of influences on how student nurses learnt to communicate and manage their emotions. For example one patient said that nurses needed both 'intelligence and the education' to enable them 'to take great care of you'. They also needed to 'follow the correct protocol when dressing my wound and to have a good bedside manner'. In other words the nurse needed to be both technically competent (she followed the right protocol) and communicative (she had a good bedside manner).

Patients identified a good nurse as someone they could trust and rely upon to give them the information they needed:

> You very quickly realize who is a good nurse … they know what they are talking about, they always come back when they say they will and clearly lay out what is going to happen to you.

The reverse situation was when patients said they were:

> …. scared to complain in case it influences the care you are given…. You might notice for example your side table is dirty but you don't want to stir things up or make things difficult for yourself. So you don't make trouble because they might not look after you …..

Two other patients had strong opinions about the emotional aspect of patient safety, stressing how feeling safe is crucial for patients when they come into hospital. One said:

> When you come into hospital you might never have been to one before, so it's a frightening experience.

The other added:

> Patient safety is about perceptions …and an absolute assurance that your decisions will not be countermanded…that your wishes will be respected at all times and in all ways whatever your situation, whether you are conscious or unconscious, whether you are elderly you need to feel that you are going to be treated as an individual with the right to decide for yourself.

They also agreed that ward managers and their influence on routines were crucial to patient safety as were adequate staffing levels:

It comes from the top and the culture within a ward. If it seems a bit rushed, it may be because they can't always determine what the staff ratio to patients will be – but you need enough staff available to give that sort of personal care on admission, to ensure that people are secure.

Students' experiences could be variable depending on staff teaching:

Staff need to get students to come to an understanding of what is best practice ... .in one ward students had been given very in-depth training and in another ward it had been completely different.

Staff also had to be knowledgeable and competent:

Sometimes I got the feeling that half the staff didn't actually know what was wrong with the patients and that I found shocking because there's somebody handing out medication from the trolley and they seemed quite unaware of their diagnoses.

But students also had to play their part and the importance of the questioning the student was highlighted:

The interest that the students showed was very high and the questions that came up afterwards – the students were probing, they were being educated, they were learning about individuality, to see the individual behind the condition.

One group of patients had been directly involved in teaching students, presenting them with 'real patients' stories' so as to help them to see the patients as individuals and not as 'medical problems'.

It's learning to see the patient as not just another medical problem, but as an individual, and having seen them as an individual, trying to fulfil their individual needs.

These patients were aware that the students' ability to give good care relied on trusting relationships, good communication, management and leadership by ward mangers to ensure their physical and emotional safety.

Summary

The 1980s

In the 1980s, the formal knowledge base of the nurse training programme at City Hospital was biomedical, but the informal knowledge base promoted a people-orientated approach to care in keeping with national ideologies. The national ideology looked for formalization of people-orientated knowledge and recognition of the nurse's unique skills, distinct from that of medicine's. At City, the local ideology promoted care as part of the 'natural' package of the nurse brought by virtue of the caring, female qualities that brought her into nursing. The local ideology was reinforced by informal knowledge and ward experience, rather than by looking at care as something that needs to be formally taught, supported and learnt.

The reason why 'nothing is really said about care' by the nurse teachers seemed to be because many of them either had doubts whether, or were unsure how, the content and teaching of nursing knowledge should differ from its traditional biomedical base. Few of them therefore used the nursing process as a conceptual means to defining an alternative approach to nursing knowledge from a biomedical one.

During sessions designated as affective/psychosocial nursing, teachers recognized the need and attempted to train students to care emotionally for patients as distinct from carrying out technical and physical tasks based on a biomedical approach to nursing. But these sessions were limited both in quantity and quality. They gave the students an occasional opportunity to describe their emotional work, but little knowledge or guidance on how to manage their feelings.

The students' own view, in the absence of an alternative model was that emotional care could not be formally taught. The psychiatric module coming at the end of their second year gave them a glimpse of an alternative perspective.

Patients held the view that, while nurses brought innate qualities essential to nursing, they also required training to strengthen them. Some patients and students also recognized that emotion management was required to induce and suppress feelings to maintain an outward appearance of calm.

My conclusion was that, at City Hospital, nursing continued to be seen as women's natural work, devalued and de-skilled because it drew its status and prestige from biomedical knowledge associated with medical techniques and procedures which treated diseases rather than people.

The 2000s

Since the completion of the first study, the two worlds of practice and formal classroom activities have become even more separate, and there has been an uncoupling of the education and clinical sectors. The formal knowledge base of nursing is prescribed by the NMC, and there is a clear acknowledgement that this must include evidence-based practice and research mediated through communication, clinical skills and competences. The nursing process as either a philosophy or work method no longer features as central to the curriculum and has been replaced by the language used in policy to promote communication, compassion, safety, equality and diversity. The Department of Health's Essence of Care benchmarks launched in 2001 were said to emphasize the 'softer aspects of care' that were key to ensuring the patient had a 'quality experience' on the one hand but provide a driver to improve quality on the other. These policy documents and a variety of Department of Health and Higher Education frameworks have been used by the NMC as a way of ensuring the nursing curriculum takes account of the main influences apparent within the two sectors. Consequently, nursing in the 2000s now finds itself squeezed between higher education and professional regulation and the potentially competing demands of government, education and the profession which have had a limiting effect on curriculum development and the content of nurse education. Nursing has little or no autonomy; rather it appears to have lost its 'internal anchors' which were apparent in the 1980s such as the hospital-based schools of nursing integrated with practice through the NHS, the nursing process as a philosophy and work method and reinforced by 'new' nursing initiatives.

The patient experience however remains a key driver and interviews with patients about patient safety confirm that for them their expectations of nursing lie with the need for good communication systems and caring based on supportive relationships between patients and nurses, and nurses and their clinical leaders. The language and structure of the curriculum may have changed, but the importance of the emotional labour of nursing remains a priority for patients and is integral as to how they feel about the quality of their hospital experience. How then are these changes perceived in the 'different world' of the ward and the student's experience of practice as a supernumerary student rather than as a member of the paid workforce and supported by a mentor rather than a ward sister? We now explore how students in the mid-2000s perceived nursing during their placements and the way in which the ward was a 'different world' from that of the 1980s.

You learn from what's wrong with the patient: defining nursing work

In the 'different world' of the 1980s, students moved through 15 clinical placements according to the medical specialities that also defined the formal content of their training.[1] At the City Hospital, as in most British teaching hospitals, the wards acquired their labels according to the speciality of the consultant physicians and surgeons who worked there, treating patients and teaching medical students. The wards were roughly divided between medicine and surgery, and then subdivided according to such specialities as oncology, neurology, gastroenterology, cardiology or orthopaedics. Specialities such as geriatrics, psychiatry, paediatrics, obstetrics and gynaecology were likely to be on separate wards and even in separate 'sister' hospitals. As the students progressed through their 15 placements, they not only changed wards but in some instances also hospitals, in order to fulfil their medically defined training requirements. The reason why they continued to see nursing as a branch of medicine thus became apparent.

One student summed up this view when she reacted to the idea that all ward experiences, irrespective of medical speciality, were of equal value because 'it's all nursing. I think it's very blind of anybody to believe that', she said, 'because you learn from what's *wrong* with the patient'. In other words, nursing for this student, like the majority of her colleagues, depended on the medical diagnosis of the patient and by association the medical speciality of the ward.

One of the drivers to undertake a follow up study was that the landscape of nursing and nurse education in the 2000s has changed so much. Nursing is no longer defined by medical diagnosis and speciality in the way described by the 1980s student. Government policy and Nursing and Midwifery Council (NMC) regulations, competences and essential skills clusters set standards and shape the structure and organization of the curriculum, and a clear distinction is drawn between the academic and practice learning environments.

Some similarities remain with students undertaking specialist modules such as obstetrics, paediatrics, care of the elderly and psychiatry, which many regard as a period away from 'mainstream' nursing, namely medicine and surgery. The difference is that now students are likely to undertake both 'mainstream' modules interspersed with specialist placements throughout their three-year programme rather than as in 1984 being concentrated in their second year.[2] However, medical and surgical specialities still tend to operate as the corner stone of clinical learning, particularly for adult nursing students.[3]

The learning environment survey undertaken in 1984 and repeated in 2007 allowed some comparisons of student perceptions that contributed to the emotional labour analysis to be made. In both surveys I wanted to find out whether there were some specialities where emotional labour was made more explicit and whether their perceptions changed at certain stages of their training. The key item 'I am happy with the experience I have had on this placement' was identified as indicative of how satisfied they felt with the learning environment.

You learn from what's wrong with the patient: how medical specialities legitimize nursing work

In this section I explore further why the student in the first study was not of the view that all ward experiences were of equal value because 'it's all nursing'.

As I talked to students in 1984 about their clinical experiences the more it became apparent that a pecking order of ward specialities existed.[4] This pecking order was not unique to the students but reflected a common societal view that valued high-tech medicine and marginalized the caretaking activities associated with caring for the elderly and chronically sick. It was also in direct contradiction with national nursing ideologies, which wanted to de-link nursing from medicine. The pecking order also reflected the role confusion experienced by students as both workers and learners. Since their formal knowledge and practice was based on medical specialities, the prestige and status afforded to certain of those specialities shaped the way in which they defined the content of their work and learning and its physical, technical or emotional components and not national nursing ideologies. The pecking order also reflected the students' shift from people-orientated nursing to a biomedical approach, described in Chapter 3. These findings are hardly surprising, but what they did show was that the new forms of nurse training promoted by the national training bodies as early as the 1950s were not sufficiently established to counter this divide.[5]

The general medical wards were lowest in the pecking order. Many of the patients were elderly and suffering from chronic conditions. Then there were the specialist medical wards such as neurology, cardiology and oncology. Thirdly, there were the surgical wards where 'you learn a completely different type of nursing from medicine, because you have to be more alert'.

At the bottom were the general medical wards where the content of the work was characterized as mostly physical. At the top were the surgical wards where the work was seen as mostly technical. In between were the specialist medical wards where the work was identified as both technical and physical and in the case of oncology, also emotional.

The psychiatric experience, coming at the end of their second year of specialities, was different from anything else the nurses experienced elsewhere in their training, because the content of their work and learning was defined only in emotional terms.

Students held low opinions about the value of their learning on some general medical wards. One student went so far as to compare it to working in a nursing home before she started training, commenting that 'I don't think I've learnt a lot more on the medical wards than I did when I was working in the nursing home'. Her judgement was based on the amount of physical care that patients required according to their age and general medical condition rather than the technical procedures required by surgical patients.

Caring for elderly patients was seen by students as '*just* having to help old people get up in the morning, get dressed and persevere with them'. Other students spoke disparagingly of elderly patients who had been admitted to the general wards for 'social' rather than 'medical' problems. A problem was defined as 'social' if patients could no longer care for themselves because of impaired function due to ageing and chronic rather than acute disease. Such patients were described as 'bed blockers', as taking up valuable space from patients in need of 'real' medical and nursing attention.[6]

This view of elderly people as 'bed blockers' is still sadly in evidence and perhaps reinforced by the pressure of NHS targets. However one student in the later study who was 'passionate' about older people's care' fiercely defended them against being negatively labelled in this way. Another student valued her experience with older people during a placement in a nursing home because she said it gave her confidence to make relationships with residents and their families which prepared her for working in the busy NHS.

Three general female wards in the earlier study were constantly cited by students as being at the bottom of the pecking order of medical specialities (and hence of learning potential), because they admitted a high percentage of elderly patients who fell into this category. The wards were described as 'heavy' because of the high physical dependency of many of the patients. At best, these wards were seen as offering 'brilliant learning experience' for first-year students because of the 'good basic experience' they offered.

Open-ended comments provided further evidence that care of the elderly, 'heavy', 'basic' or 'routine' work were described as valuable to learning almost exclusively by first-year students. At the other end of the spectrum, routine/basic work generated by elderly and/or physically dependent patients was seen as least valuable irrespective of year of training with the care of elderly people when viewed as a speciality being particularly unpopular with senior students (see: Companion website, Appendix E, Smith 1992).

It appeared therefore that students' perception of the ward learning environment depended to some extent on an interaction between their year of training and the specialty of their placement which was influenced by their view that some wards and specialities were more appropriate to their learning at different stages of their three-year programme.

In 2007, there did not seem to be a significant variation in student satisfaction when analysed in relation to their year of study nor according to the university where they were registered. The finding that neither year of study nor university made an overall difference to their perception of satisfaction at any point in their three-year programme may have been because they were allocated to both general and specialist placements throughout. It was decided therefore to combine the two items, 'happy with experience' and 'learning opportunities' to indicate 'net satisfaction' and to analyse it in the context of placement speciality to see whether there was any variation as there had been in 1984.

On scrutinizing the ratings of net satisfaction against placement speciality, it was possible to observe that the students (92%) appeared to be the most satisfied with their intensive care placements while satisfaction with their placements in the Accident and Emergency department, surgery, community/primary health care, acute medicine and mental health, were all high at around 70%. The students appeared to be least satisfied with their placements in the care of older people (46%) and care homes (30%). These trends were similar to the findings of the first survey and suggested that present day students expressed similar preferences to their predecessors in that they were more satisfied with their placements in acute and/or specialist settings compared with their placements in the care of older people where the net satisfaction in these placements, particularly in care homes, dropped dramatically.

Placements in acute and specialist settings on the other hand offered technical nursing and medical knowledge, investigations and treatments that students saw as particularly valuable to their learning (see: Companion website, Appendix E, Tables E3 and E5, Smith 1992).

Students in the first study learnt very quickly to distinguish between the work of general and specialist medical wards. For example, one student, less than six months into training, compared the 'heavy' routine work of her first allocation to the specialist neurological ward where she was now assigned. 'It's unlike most other medical wards' she said in a thrilled voice 'because there are loads of different illnesses and multiple sclerosis and all that and people coming in for tests and lumbar punctures and things'. In her excitement she saw neurology as exotic diseases and tests rather than uncertainty, unpleasant symptoms and long-term suffering for patients and their families.

Experience on surgical wards was predominantly seen as learning about techniques: patients were much more likely to have intravenous infusions, urinary catheters, surgical dressings, suction and other types of surgical drainage than their counterparts on the medical wards. On the surgical wards, there were a variety of techniques that students could observe being performed: changing dressings or intravenous infusion bags, inserting catheters or removing surgical drains and stitches. As one student observed 'You can learn from watching techniques being done'. Another student was excited by learning to care for surgical patients with a very quick turnover, and to manage emergencies such as plummeting blood pressures or haemorrhaging wounds.

Interestingly, in the 2000s, the expression 'a very quick turnover' has become the predominant feature of the current learning environment with ward managers describing the clinical areas as 'so very busy, busier than in the past'. They attributed this increased 'busyness' to government policy which was having a direct effect on practice and students' learning experience. Even students were very aware of government policy and mentioned that they learnt 'a lot about it' in class.

Two practice educators (PEs) who were responsible for organizing students' clinical support listed the policies which in their view were putting both students and trained staff under new pressures. These policies included Essence of Care, National Service Frameworks (NSF), National Institute of Clinical Excellence (NICE) guidelines, Clinical Risk, the four-hour wait in Accident and Emergency and the six-week surgery waiting times. Many of these policies were evident in the content of the students' formal curriculum as discussed in Chapter 3.

The PEs concluded that:

> The effects of these policies are felt down to the grassroots and the students will be well aware of these targets. There is constantly a pressure on empty beds. Students will be aware of the constant telephone calls to check the bed state and the number of empty beds so that patients can be moved from A&E within the four hour target.

The educators also described the impact of a number of initiatives to deal with 'throughput' of patients. One such initiative involved setting up a Clinical Decision Unit (next to the A&E department) which allowed patients to be transferred out of A&E into a 'holding bay' within four hours of admission (in order to meet the four-hour target). Here patients were assessed and observed until they were either deemed ready for discharge or in need of admission requiring that a bed be 'found' for them. They would then stay on the ward until they were ready for discharge, when they would be transferred to a 'Discharge Lounge' in order to vacate their bed for the next patient. They would then wait in the 'Discharge

Lounge' elsewhere in the hospital for transport to take them home and/or for their drugs to be dispensed by the pharmacy.

Another consequence of these new 'speed-up' policies was that during their hospital stay patients could 'get shipped all around the hospital' as part of throughput i.e. 'keeping them moving through the acute wards'. The educators commented that fast throughput was 'a nightmare' for infection control (the beds were always full to capacity which could have a deleterious effect on hygiene).[7] It also meant that patients might get moved inappropriately, which was not necessarily in the best interests of their welfare.

The educators concluded that:

> In this fast pace and patient turnover, learning (other than observing) becomes difficult for both the mentor and the student. Especially when statutory training days[8] are difficult to organize to ensure safe levels of knowledge among trained staff'.

A student's comment in the 2007 survey confirmed this view. She described her experiences on her last placement as stressful because of:

> ... under-staffing and a lack of time for the trained staff to sit down and actually address the learning needs of the students, including having the time to sit down and go through the paperwork. It was often 5 minutes snatched in the middle of the ward.

Some ward managers were concerned that the students were unprepared for the 'quick and fast' environment of their placements and that their lecturers needed to equip them to deal with the changes in hospital organization. On their part, the lecturers were aware that the ward environment could be busy and stressful for both students and staff which could make learning difficult.

One student described how she was kept 'very busy' in a day surgery unit with a high turnover, where 'short stay' patients were expected to be 'out' of the unit within twenty-three hours. In the immediate post operative period the patients needed half-hourly post operative observations, which the student described as 'difficult' but manageable because she 'kept up ... by learning to do things faster'.

This student demonstrated resourcefulness in managing her learning in the 'quick and fast' conditions of the NHS.

One consequence of the 'quick and fast' conditions such as 'high turnover' and 'speed up' is that a sharp division of labour has emerged that differentiates between technical nursing (drains, dressings and drugs) and personal care in order to get the work done. Technical nursing is regarded as the preserve of qualified nurses in their new managerial and specialist clinical nursing roles while personal care is considered to be the primary responsibility of HCAs. Often the students reported feeling caught in the middle especially in their third year if they were overloaded with giving personal care rather than learning technical nursing. This was because they equated personal care with caring[9] rather than nursing and therefore did not prepare them for their future roles.

In the 1980s, when students were apprentices they would expect to give the full spectrum of care comprising technical, physical and affective tasks which they related to their stage of training rather than to a specific role within the division of labour of the nursing workforce.

In the 2000s they identified their learning according to how they described and identified workforce roles and relationships among themselves, qualified nurses and HCAs rather than distinguishing between specialities as a way of learning about specific techniques.

During fieldwork one senior third year student expressed her concern at the end of a physically demanding shift exclaiming 'you know what am I doing here and not even drugs yet?! What have I done today? Caring not nursing and another shift wasted!'

The concern that caring may not be nursing and therefore not valuable for learning continued to be expressed by students throughout their three-year programme rather than identifying medical knowledge as a primary source of learning.

Their lecturers were concerned that the students learnt the 'essential skills' of nursing and described this as a dilemma in terms of the individuals from whom they should be learning them.

As one lecturer explained:

Students are no longer the workforce providing basic care. Health Care Assistants are doing this, so students no longer seek to do basic care. They seek to instruct others to do it rather than have a lifetime of doing it themselves. The students see that the role of the staff nurse is the management of care, administration, organization and communication outside the ward.

A student in a questionnaire comment reported that:

Being treated as an HCA on a daily basis was preventing me learning as much as I could learn on the placement.

The student's comment reflects one lecturer's concern that the students did not have role models among nursing leaders who gave hands on care. She said:

Leaders of nursing should supervise care and you need to give care to know how to supervise it.

Another lecturer referred to the development of specialist nursing within the nursing workforce which potentially deprived students of new role models on a routine basis in the wards. The lecturer explained how these 'new' clinical leaders of nursing, many of whom worked within multidisciplinary teams, needed to teach as they worked with both students and qualified staff:

> Role models are needed for students to identify what contribution nursing makes to the multi disciplinary team – specialist nurses have deskilled general nurses and students need exposure to all nursing leadership roles. Specialist nurses need to see pre-registration teaching as part of their remit as well as working and teaching registered nurses within the speciality.

As well as changes in workforce roles, one student, also quoted in Chapter 6, explained that the experience of undertaking care work in the calmer context of a residential home had equipped her for the 'busyness' of the NHS. She described how in the home she had learnt confidence through meeting people, making relationships with them and getting to know them. Now she was undertaking her surgical placement, she could see how these skills had given her confidence to cope with the faster pace and higher turnover of an acute hospital ward. This student's view of the value to learning of being placed in a nursing home, contrasted strongly with the student in the first study who was very dismissive of the 'heavy' routine work on both general medical wards and nursing homes.

Recognizing emotion work

The 1980s

In the 1980s study I wanted to identify those specialities where emotional work was explicitly recognized. I found at that time that it was only in the oncology wards in the students' 'general' experience that the nature of their work and associated learning was unequivocally described as having an explicit emotional component. One reason for this was the medical legitimization of emotion work within the speciality.[10] One student described how it 'began to dawn' on her when she was on an oncology ward at the end of her first year 'the amount of psychological needs that people have'. 'Until then' she said 'I hadn't realized what people's needs are when they are in hospital'. Another student described the oncology ward as the place where she learnt about 'human emotion', because 'you see the patients in such a lot of trouble'. She also described the work in terms of oncological techniques and specialist nursing. The medical legitimization of emotion work within oncology was reinforced by the powerful image of cancer in society as a symbol of suffering and death, vividly described by Susan Sontag (1983) in her essay on 'Illness as Metaphor'.

I was interested by another student's perspectives, which illustrated how a medical speciality served to legitimize nursing's emotional as well as technical components by comparing her experiences on ophthalmology with an oncology ward. She said of the ophthalmology ward:

> I would have liked to have been taught more about 'the eyes' really on that ward. I mean it's quite fun chatting to the patients but the actual nursing is boring. Anybody can bathe an eye. But I dare say if you are an ophthalmologist in a clinic it's different. It's more a doctor's thing than a nurse's from my point of view.

I then asked her what she thought of as a 'nurse's thing'. She replied: 'Maybe oncology is much more of a nurse's world because there is so much more psychological care'.

In other words, this student perceived oncology patients as generating 'psychological care' as part of the work, whereas patients with eye problems were merely 'quite fun' to chat to.

On the other hand, this student also suggests that psychological care associated with oncology, is more a 'nurse's world' than a speciality such as 'ophthalmology', which she sees as being more dependent on medical skills.

Yet in the ward survey, only 15 per cent of comments identified the emotional components of nursing (e.g. care of terminal patients and their relatives, talking to them and controlling their pain) as valuable to learning (see: Companion website, Appendix E, Table E4, Smith 1992). Students were more likely to identify these experiences when they were allocated to oncology wards, even though patients on all medical wards might be in pain, suffer from cancer, die or need nurses to talk to.

In Chapter 3 I describe the importance of the psychiatric nursing module for making students more aware of the 'psychological side' of patient care, and this is illustrated by one student's insights when feelings ran high for both patients and staff.

> If there was an intense staff interaction, say when the patient's being very aggressive and you get upset. It would be put directly to someone in charge. Everything would stop. There would be a discussion. It wouldn't just be 'what should we do about this?' First of all the trained staff would start on you. 'How does this upset you? Are you sure you feel alright? This plan of action isn't working with this patient. Let's go and talk to them and let them know'.

The focus of work on the psychiatric ward was clearly defined around relationships and feelings and how to manage them systematically. The person in charge would stop 'everything' to discuss a patient care issue and how it affected the nurses. This approach was very much in contrast to most general wards, where (with the possible exception of oncology) even at that time patient care was organized to 'keep going' in order to manage high turnover, technical procedures and 'heavy' physical work, irrespective of how the students felt. But the urgency of the work, and the power and persuasiveness of the image of acute hospital nursing, was not only felt by students. A committed psychiatric nurse and teacher told me that, even after years of working in a psychiatric hospital, she experienced a fleeting feeling on entering the corridors of City, busy with nurses and porters escorting patients on trolleys and wheelchairs and intravenous drips, that this was 'real' nursing and not the emotional labour of the psychiatric wards.

The 2000s

In the current health service patients' length of hospital stay is much shorter than it was in the 1980s. Students therefore have less time to get to know the patients, coupled with the fact that their time spent on wards is much reduced in most placements. The social cohesion of spending eight intensive weeks on the ward as part of the workforce no longer exists in the same way throughout training. Furthermore the diversity and multiculturalism of the contemporary workforce, and patient and student profile was recognized during interviews but not taken account of in the ward environment, partly because of 'busyness' but also because of the lack of formal training and organizational support to address these issues which in turn could create a potential barrier to student learning.

Additional barriers to learning such as students' emotional preparedness for the type and pace of work as well as their emotional maturity when caring for sick and dying patients were also identified. While there was an awareness that students could be overwhelmed not only by the busy nature of the clinical areas but also by the nature of the work, opportunities for reflection when dealing with difficult emotional situations across the range did not appear to be routine practice.

PEs in one site described why 'emotional preparedness' for clinical areas was important and discussed the need for appropriate placements to match the students' stage of training and to fit in with their prior placement experience. One PE described the following situation:

> I had a student who was at the end of her first year. It was her first time in a hospital setting and she had never taken any one to the toilet or given anyone a urinal. Well she felt stupid so she didn't like to ask how to do it.

This student was experiencing the 'culture shock' described in Chapter 3 of students returning or even being placed for the first time on acute 'mainstream' wards following their community nursing placements. The PEs concluded on the basis of this example that acute care placements were not suitable for a first year student; 'Cardiology' as a first acute speciality placement was described as 'too technical for them'. Neither was an acute care placement deemed suitable for those second-year students who had come directly from having only had prior community or nursing home experience. Such students were described as 'being frightened' or 'out of their depth' when they were placed in an acute setting.

When the feelings don't fit

The category 'when the feelings don't fit' was originally derived from students' survey responses, which showed that in the 1984 study the nature of the work on all 12 medical wards generated a range of feelings within the students that could have been contained by appropriate handling or emotion management by the trained staff as exemplified by the approach used on the psychiatric wards. When their feelings didn't fit with what was expected of them they experienced stress and anxiety as rated on a four-point scale from 3.0 (frequently experienced) to 0 (never experienced) during their eight-week allocation. The average scores for the 12 wards ranged from 2.24 to 1.44 (see Companion website, Appendix E, Table E6 (a), Smith 1992). No ward achieved a 'zero' stress rating, i.e. anxiety or stress was 'never' not experienced by students as a group on any one ward. Four wards were shown to have high stress ratings that were statistically significant compared with the others (see: Companion website, Appendix E, Table E6 (b), Smith 1992). Two of these wards were oncology wards, and the other two had very demanding workloads for different reasons. One ward was a 'heavy' female medical ward with low staffing levels, resulting in students feeling frustration and guilt because of being unable to get through the work, and the other was a male medical ward with a high turnover of acutely ill patients.

Students were also asked to comment on the causes of stress and anxiety on the wards. The nature and volume of the work, ward speciality, type of patients and low staffing levels were frequently implicated. For example, one student found the speciality of oncology 'imposed stress on me as a person' while another student experienced stress, physical tiredness and depression because of feeling unable to get the work done on a 'heavy female medical ward'. She implied that her feelings were partly to do with the type of work generated by dependent elderly female patients, but also with the lack of staff to carry out the work. Dying patients were mentioned as causes of stress particularly on the oncology wards, but also on two other wards (gastroenterology and cardiology). Fear of patients suffering from cardiac arrests created stress and anxiety for students on the two cardiology wards, even though such incidents rarely happened.

In 2007 just over two-thirds of the questionnaire respondents indicated that they had experienced some degree of stress or anxiety during their current or most recent placement while the remaining third said they 'hardly ever' or 'never' experienced stress or anxiety. These findings may suggest that contemporary students' feelings were more effectively managed than those of their predecessors. I also explored whether there was an association between the students' perceptions of stress and anxiety and how they rated their satisfaction on the item 'I am happy with my placement experience'. An association appeared to exist in that when students indicated they either strongly agreed or agreed they were 'happy' with their placement the majority of them (91%) reported they had rarely experienced stress or anxiety. When students reported they *had experienced stress and anxiety during their placements* this percentage dropped to just over two thirds (68%), suggesting that stress and anxiety played a part in how they rated whether they were happy or not with their experience.

As in the first study I also wanted to examine the survey findings for associations between levels of stress and anxiety and placement speciality. Nearly three quarters of the contemporary respondents experienced some degree of stress and anxiety if their most recent placement had been in the Accident and Emergency department or the acute medical, surgical and intensive care wards compared with community/primary health care placements where over half the respondents 'hardly ever or never' experienced stress or anxiety. Oncology was not distinguished as a discrete speciality as it had been in 1984, although students described the stress and anxiety associated with caring for dying patients and bereaved relatives during their placements both in terms of the nature of the experience and the support required.[11] Satisfaction with some specialities most associated with stress and anxiety was high (e.g. intensive care, accident and emergency). Clearly stress and anxiety alone did not determine levels of satisfaction within a placement even though the two were significantly related; it may even suggest that in some circumstances supporting students to manage the stress of caring for critically ill patients can play a positive role in the learning process, a finding suggested by students allocated to hospices.

Other reasons for feeling stressed or anxious, which students described in their open-ended comments included supernumerary status not being a reality in practice; being used as a 'spare pair of hands' or as an 'HCA'; 'lack of time for teaching and learning' because of high workload and inadequate staffing levels; lack of continuity in placement (being switched around from team to team or location to location); and having no time to build up relationships with trained staff.

These comments were further substantiated by their responses to the questionnaire items. For example, there was a statistically significant relationship between how often students expressed stress and anxiety in relation to the provision of an atmosphere 'which is good to work in' by sister and trained staff. Ward atmosphere appeared to be a mitigating factor in that when they perceived the ward atmosphere positively, fewer of them (56%) indicated they had experienced stress and anxiety compared with those students (92%) who perceived it negatively. On a related item a large majority of respondents (68%) agreed or strongly agreed that 'on this ward sister and trained nurses work as a team with learners'. When this item was correlated with their perceptions of stress and anxiety, 92% of those who rated it negatively had experienced some level of stress or anxiety on their current or most recent placement compared to just 54% who rated team working positively, indicating that lack of team working was associated with higher levels of anxiety and stress. These findings strongly suggest that a positive ward atmosphere and team work makes an important contribution to the students' emotional wellbeing.

Given that supernumerary status was one of the big changes to have been introduced since the first study when students had been regarded as part of the workforce the questionnaire item 'The workload does not interfere with teaching or learning' was identified as an indicator of 'supernumerary' status and substantiated by open-ended comments. Indeed a positive association was found when students' perception of their supernumerary status (i.e. the workload did not interfere with teaching or learning) was correlated with the two indicator items of placement satisfaction i.e. they were 'happy with the experience' and their 'learning'.

The mentor was identified as playing an important role in their learning and teaching. In particular the students valued them being easily accessible and supportive throughout their placements. When this was not the case students said that they felt more stressed and anxious. For example PEs reported that student learning 'other than observing' was difficult, because although *officially* expected to be 'supernumerary' during their placements, they were *unofficially* expected to work as part of the workforce when the wards were busy. Students, for their part, demonstrated resourcefulness in the face of these demands in managing their supernumerary status to work as a member of the workforce helped by supportive mentors who were 'always around'.

I also looked at the students' perceptions of their supernumerary status and specialities, and they appeared to most strongly agree that the workload did not interfere with teaching and learning in intensive care and community/primary health placements. In these two specialities students were most likely to agree or strongly agree that 'trained nurses teach as they work with learners'. Workload was perceived to interfere with teaching and learning to varying degrees in all the other specialities. The most interference with teaching and learning was perceived to be in mental health, care homes, surgery, the Accident and Emergency department, care of older people and acute medicine. On the related item 'trained nurses teach as they work with learners' the students were more likely to disagree with this statement for these specialities, especially in the care homes.

In 2007, a third year student described how her lecturers encouraged students to be assertive and self-empowered and to act as agents of change, yet her experience of the NHS and nursing was hierarchical and bullying and she said 'I feel like I'm in the playground again'.

Students in both surveys rated patient care as being good overall in their placements, and the scores on this dimension continued to be among the most favourable (see: Companion website, Appendix E, Table E7, Smith 1992 and Methodological Appendix II, Smith 2012).

In the 2007 survey, when it came to explaining the relationship between patient care and student learning a number of correlations were examined on items such as 'patients receive the best attention and nursing care', 'this was a good placement for student learning' and 'trained nurses teach as they work with learners' which were all positively associated. In terms of specialities and perceptions of care delivery, intensive care, the accident and emergency department and community/primary health care were rated the most positively compared with care of older people and care home placements, which they perceived as having lower standards of care delivery.

These findings suggest that patients receive the best attention and nursing care in specialities where students are satisfied with their learning opportunities. These findings are similarly related to the contact they perceive they have with trained nurses (and their mentors) as they work. The three specialities they rate highest in this respect – intensive care, accident and emergency, and community/primary health care all require the input and support of trained nurses alongside students, whereas the care of older people and care home placements are not regarded as requiring input from qualified nurses since the care is perceived as 'personal' and 'general' rather than 'technical' and 'specialist'.

When the scores for each of the four items of the dimension students' perceptions of patient care were combined to give a mean score of 3.64, the score obtained was lower than the mean score obtained by their 1984 counterparts which was 4.16. One reason for this lower score might be because contemporary students are considered to be supernumerary and therefore do not regard themselves as part of the workforce nor directly responsible for patient care. The students in 1984 were clearly regarded as the frontline workforce and saw themselves as the ones who 'care more because there are more of us!' – now the role of frontline care has become the primary domain of HCAs.

In the 1984 survey, the students' higher scores for patient care suggest two things: firstly that as the principal care givers, they were rating their own care and secondly that, despite understaffing and high patient workloads, they felt they were giving patients good care. This assumption and related evidence further suggests that even when the 'feelings don't fit', students laboured both physically and emotionally to care for the patients by suppressing their own feelings. The following comment by a student responding to the 2007 survey suggests they also laboured in this way when:

> There was too much work on the ward and not enough staff which meant that I was not able to give the time to care for the patients as much as I would have liked to without the feeling of being hurried.

This student clearly saw frontline care as part of her remit but as a consequence of a high workload and insufficient staff unable to give the time required to care for patients in the way she would have liked 'without the feel of being hurried.'

Returning to the 1984 survey a further example of the way in which students undertook emotional labour 'when the feelings don't fit' was revealed in the following comment by a third-year student who 'found patients frustrating'. She was working on an oncology ward and explained that she did not really want to be there, because her mother had died of cancer. The student found the female oncology patients 'frustrating and often unwilling to help themselves'. The comment suggests that little attention was paid to this student's individual needs, since neither the trained nor the tutorial staff appeared to be aware of her particular situation and/or feelings related to her mother's death.

That the students felt deeply about themselves, the patients and their work is apparent in all these descriptions. But in the 1980s the way in which the work was defined according to medical criteria set the feeling rules of the general wards, which in turn determined that the students kept their feelings to themselves.

Even an oncology ward could not accommodate the range of feelings experienced by students, especially when they related to their personal histories. When feelings were not legitimized by the feeling rules of the ward, the students felt stressed or anxious for feeling them. They therefore engaged in emotion work to present a different emotional self in the public arena of the ward.

One student, who clearly recognized that nursing work went beyond the boundaries of medical specialities, described the wards at City Hospital as being 'so keyed up to a certain specialty, not nursing care-wise but the doctors who are orientated in that way. That's what they're good at and that's what they deal with. And when you get a patient who isn't their sort of norm then they do tend to be at a bit of a loss'. We can postulate that when the doctors 'are at a bit of a loss', it is then that they 'dump' patients on nurses.

We also saw that students received limited formal training or support to deal with emotionally charged situations, and few classroom or ward discussions gave them the opportunity to discuss their feelings systematically, both the positive and negative things which they felt about themselves and their patients.

It was not surprising, therefore, that there were certain types of patients that students preferred to nurse than others, and 'liking' someone not only facilitated good interpersonal relationships but helped their learning. As one student put it, 'You learn from the patients and you adapt to their different characters especially the patients you like the best'.

This view of 'liking' the patient links up with student perspectives on 'being nice to patients' and the need to undertake emotional labour, especially when the 'feelings don't fit'. Students previously quoted in Chapter 2 recognized that, although they were expected to 'be nice' to everyone, there were certain conditions under which this was not possible. They expected reciprocity from patients. This view was expressed about Mr Bear, an elderly patient who had recently been discharged home. A student recalled: 'Mr Bear looked so happy when he was discharged. He was very grateful and so easy to nurse; he was a lovely man. His wife said "He always said to me how good you nurses were"'. Investing emotional labour was clearly easier with 'grateful' patients like the 'lovely' Mr Bear.[12]

Patient feedback was equally important to students in 2007 as we saw in previous chapters and the little things continued to make a difference, like remembering a patient's wedding anniversary, asking people whether they were 'alright' to find out whether they 'slept okay' or had 'any worries', and for older people making sure they wore their hearing aid right up to the moment of being transferred to the operating room and helping another elderly patient with her meals.

There are some patients you'd rather nurse than others: issues of age, gender and race – then and now

In 1984 I concluded that the wards at the bottom of the students' pecking order of 'good' nursing experience admitted a high percentage of elderly female patients with general medical conditions. These patients were rated as generating a high physical workload with poor learning potential.

One student said that one of the reasons why she preferred nursing younger patients was that she found she had a lot more consideration for their feelings. I suppose you shouldn't have, she added guiltily, but you've got to do so much more for the elderly than for younger patients. By this she meant that the physical demands of working with the elderly left little time for considering their individual feelings. But she also felt that she had more in common with patients in their thirties than the patients of her grandparents' generation.

Part of the reason for the unpopularity of elderly women patients was because their toileting requirements were seen to generate such physically demanding work. Elderly men could use urinals either sitting in a chair or lying in bed. The urinals were kept in a wire hanger on the side of their beds, so many of them could help themselves when necessary.

However, elderly women had to be helped on to bedpans or commodes which were stored in the sluice. Each time they wanted to use the bedpan or commode they had to ring for the nurse. She then had to help the patient to the bathroom or bring the commode or the bedpan to the bedside. The curtains then had to be drawn and the patient helped on to either. When the patient was ready, she was helped off and made comfortable. All this took a lot of time, especially if up to ten patients on a ward needed to be assisted in this way.

It is interesting that patients frequently commented on the 'endless patience' students had 'with the old ones'. Knowing as I did how negatively students often felt about nursing elderly patients, this suggested that they worked on these negative feelings to appear as if they had 'endless patience'. Similarly there were students in 2007 passionately committed to the care of older people who gave them their time and attention. The encouragement of their mentors who set the tone was very important as described in Chapter 6, when elderly distressed and sometimes demented patients were prepared for emergency surgery with soothing words and extra oxygen.

The gender aspects of the 2007 study were implicit rather than explicit, and gender was used as a unit of analysis in relation to students rather than patients. The language of the curriculum emphasized the importance of gender as a key element of diversity and equal opportunities. Furthermore the student body was older overall than in 1984 with a larger percentage of mature students who were married and/or had children. Many of them had also worked as HCAs prior to undertaking their nurse training, and some of them were still working in these roles to supplement their bursaries. Overall, given their profile it was likely that that more students in the 2007 group were familiar with the issues of giving personal care and caring for older dependent people than the City hospital cohorts. In addition they had undertaken a range of personal care work both for their own children and elderly relatives. Some students attributed feelings of stress and anxiety to the challenge of balancing the demands of their many roles which they described as parent, partner, student on campus and placement, and in some cases paid employee. Although the majority of commentators were women, one male student also pointed out that given 11% of the nursing workforce were men, they could also face these challenges.

In 1984 gender was analysed in relation to the students' views on the patients' gender, which they related not only to the physical component of their work, but also to their social relations. Many of their expectations and interpretations were based on gender stereotypes. For example, two students on the eve of their first ward allocation thought they would prefer working with men because:

> Women are fussy. They expect a 'hotel service' as if they were on holiday. Men are more considerate of nurses. They've got more pride to get on their feet and they don't like women doing things.

Another student, also at the beginning of training, thought it would be easier to work on a men's ward:

> Because they are more encouraging than women and they like being fussed over. Women don't. They feel their independence has gone as mothers and they say 'You should be able to do it [nursing work] better'.

Following her first ward experience of nursing women, this student thought that her predictions had been confirmed:

> I think that men would be more grateful. A lot of the women like to be independent. They don't like you telling them what to do. They say 'I could teach you nurses a few things'. Some of them expect you to do everything and they don't say 'please' and 'thank you'.

Another student thought that women 'called out for you. Men are more sort of passive and far more independent'.

These comments show the issue of nursing as women's work. Female patients as wives and mothers were seen as having some expertise in the type of activities that nurses undertook, the tasks described as women's attributes (Ungerson 1983b). Nurses felt threatened but also resented having to do things for female patients which the patients, as women, usually did for others. They were harder on the women because of this, and expected more gratitude from them. They also expected women to 'take advantage' of their stay in hospital by seeing it as time off from their domestic tasks. Many nurses also expected that, because of this, women patients would also 'take advantage' of them.

The effects of gender on nurse–patient relationships in long-stay geriatric hospitals are discussed by Evers (1981b). She suggested that the 'mothering' model adopted by many of the nurses in caring for their elderly patients in her study was more suited to male patients, since men are used to being serviced in their domestic lives by women. Women, on the other hand, were not used to being serviced by anybody and wanted to maintain their independence.

Although I found in my 1980s study that the outcome was similar to Evers' findings, the students did not articulate their role as a 'mothering' one, but associated their 'non-technical' activities with the basic skills they acquired in their first few weeks of nursing. Their emotional work was part of the package they brought with them as white middle-class women, which included a range of gender stereotypes which shaped their relationships with male and female patients.

A third-year Student preferred nursing men for the following reasons:

I just find men easier to talk to a lot of the time and they have got a different idea of hospitals. Women can almost expect to be waited on as if they've come in for a rest. Men want to get out of hospital as quickly as possible and they just want to be as independent as possible.

Other students found women easier to talk to because of being women. One nurse found that women were 'more open to discussion' whereas 'men see you just as a nurse'. Another student preferred nursing women because she thought that 'old men touch you up'.

One of the few male nurse interviewees had the following views on nursing male and female patients:

Patients react differently to male nurses. Women appreciate having a man about the place. It's just a change in atmosphere perhaps. You look upon the technicalities in much the same way, like dressings and getting your drips through on time. In the more social aspects I think probably women talk more easily to women. I think perhaps men talk more easily to women as well, although I think it varies a lot.

These comments illustrate that nurses recognized that gender was important in terms of their social relations and ability to talk with each other. Sexuality was only alluded to and requires further exploration. However, students talked at some length about dealing with violent patients, usually men, and the underlying sexuality implicit in their accounts emerged. The accounts provide further evidence of the lack of opportunity to discuss their feelings systematically, both positive and negative, which they felt about themselves and their patients and how to handle them.

The reactions and perceptions of the contemporary students reflected their different life experiences and 'mature' age profile than those of their predecessors.

When emotional labour is the work: the case of violent patients

The 1980s

Tracy, a student at the end of her allocation to the ward with the highest stress/anxiety rating of all 12 medical wards, was in a low physical and emotional state when I interviewed her. She was losing her voice because of a severe respiratory infection. Many of the nurses had been sick, she said, which she put down to the stressful conditions on the ward.

I had worked on that ward a few months prior to the interview. The workload was unpredictable because the physicians admitted many of their patients from the hospital's accident and emergency department. Being in the centre of the inner city, many of the patients who were admitted were young men who were drug users and who had overdosed. Apart from their precarious medical conditions in the initial stages of their admission, they could be complicated people to relate to: charming, manipulative and needing their drugs. Part of their rehabilitation was to try to convince them that they needed to be referred to a drug treatment centre. The nurses were on the front line, negotiating the doctors' instructions with the patients. A number of factors affected these negotiations, not least that the nurses and patients were part of the same generation.

Tracy described to me how one such patient who had been on the ward during her allocation had created a lot of stress for her personally. Having recovered from his overdose, the patient, who was over six feet tall, wandered about the ward clad only in his underpants. 'I found this behaviour very sexually suggestive and potentially violent', she said, 'I think partly because of his size. After all I'm only five foot and he towered over me.'

She explained that the doctors offered the patient psychiatric help, but he refused it. After that she said, 'they kept away from him as much as possible. In the end I couldn't go near him either'. Tracy was very upset that she had felt this way, and was unable to justify her withdrawal, even though the doctors had 'kept away from him' also. 'I learnt something about myself she said – I felt I had failed. Never before did I realize that there were certain patients I just couldn't cope with'.

While I was a participant observer on another ward, I observed another student, Mary, confronting a similar situation. The patient in question was Jay, a man in his forties, admitted with episodes of confusion, aggression and violent outbursts. The cause was unclear. He was a professional soldier, and there was a suggestion that his behaviour was a reaction to the stress of being in a war zone. He was tall and good looking and looked every inch the part of a hero in a war film. But there the stereotypical gallantry ended. He would wander off the ward, and any attempts at restraint precipitated aggressive and threatening behaviour. He was particularly confused at night. Two student nurses, 21 years old, were expected to take charge of Jay, along with 20 other patients at least six of whom were acutely ill. On the last night of a seven-night stretch, Mary reported sick. The staff nurse told me she was not surprised. 'I heard Mary talking to Jay this morning', she said, 'and her voice was cracking'.

When Mary came back the following week she told me how upset she'd felt over Jay's behaviour. 'We had a lot of sick patients', she said, 'and yet we had to watch that Jay didn't wander off the ward during the night. And you were never sure how he might react to you. We had absolutely no help from the doctors, although the night sisters were quite supportive. I wanted to say to Jay "Look here mate stop messing about" but I felt that I couldn't'.

When I asked her why that was, she said that it was because that was not the way one was expected to talk to patients, irrespective of how you felt. Besides, she didn't know how Jay would react.

For Mary, like Tracy, the costs were high of maintaining emotional labour when confronted by a potentially violent young male patient. Tracy withdrew her labour by avoiding the patient, but felt she had failed. Mary suppressed feelings of what she really wanted to say to the patient, but reported sick, the strain having been heard in her voice by a staff nurse on the previous shift.

The 2000s

In the recent study students did not give specific examples of encounters with 'violent' patients, nor did we observe such encounters during our fieldwork. However, in the NHS annual staff surveys, respondents now report high incidents of violence and abuse, and some specialities are regarded as particularly susceptible such as accident and emergency departments and the acute mental health wards. As mentioned previously, staff are required to undertake annual updating programmes in manual handling, health and safety and if working in these vulnerable areas restraining techniques for violent patients.

Studies of violence in the National Health Service (NHS) have found significant levels of colleague-on-colleague bullying (Quine 1999) but also of aggression on the part of patients towards healthcare professionals. The latest report on staff in the UK NHS by the Health Care Commission (Health Care Commission 2008) found that 23% of NHS staff reported being bullied by patients, 18% by patients' relatives, 8% by managers and 13% by colleagues. Paradoxically, although the majority of staff knew how to report such episodes, a substantial minority never did so. This finding confirmed Einarsen's (2004) proposal that the culture of the workplace acts as a form of filter through which a range of behaviours come to be accepted or even tolerated, despite the fact that most employees experience a high degree of role conflict when they observe aggressive behaviour and report a poor quality of environment in these circumstances.

Dispelling the stereotypes: issues of race

The 1980s

Students described their preference for nursing certain patients on the basis of age and gender stereotypes, but not race. It would not have been acceptable for the City type of nurse (i.e. white and middle-class) in the 'service of others' to express racial prejudice publicly. While I was a participant observer, however, I found that racial stereotypes emerged as an important issue from time to time in a predominantly white middle-class environment. The City Hospital was located in the inner city, with an ethnically diverse population. The majority of patients admitted to the hospital, however, were referred from outside the district. Most of them were white and middle-class, and not representative of the local population. Student contact with black patients was therefore relatively infrequent, as was the discussion of ethnic and racial diversity in their training programme, except for one of their assessment criteria described as 'awareness of patient's cultural needs'. Thus once again students were expected to meet patients' so-called cultural needs without discussing what this meant or being adequately prepared to do so. At that time, thinking among educators for a multi-racial Britain, for example, was critical of subsuming race and ethnicity under the relatively innocuous term 'culture'.[13] During their ward experiences, therefore, students were exposed to racial stereotyping without being offered any alternative perspectives with which to challenge them.

Take Miss Baxter, suffering from Parkinson's disease, who was a large black woman in her sixties and described predictably by the ward staff as a 'big black mama'. Miss Baxter, like many patients of her age and condition, snored loudly at night, and many of her neighbouring patients described her among themselves as an 'animal'. The staff and students were aware of the offensive way in which Miss

Baxter was referred to, but did not articulate it as a racist stereotype (as clearly it was), nor do anything to dispel it among the patients.

Once Miss Baxter's behaviour won the nurses' approval, she acquired another set of stereotypes during the ward handovers where she was described as 'ever such a nice lady' and 'very pleasant and smiling'. Weren't 'big black mamas' supposed to be smiling? Thus any racial stereotyping by either nurses or patients was left unchallenged and without appropriate consciousness raising, to be reproduced, potentially, at a later date by students.

The 2000s

In the 2000s issues of race, gender and sexual orientation are much more visible in policy and public life, with attention given to the promotion of equity and diversity supported by official documents published by the NHS, other public bodies and reflected in the students' curriculum described in Chapter 3.

The adoption of the language of equity and diversity is one small step towards confronting racism but as a contemporary study to explore the experiences faced by overseas nurses showed, discrimination still exists (Smith et al. 2006). The number of students who are from black and ethnic minority backgrounds is still relatively small. As presented in Chapter 2, the Nursing and Midwifery Admissions Service (NMAS) data suggest that 77% of nursing entrants describe themselves as 'White' or 'White British'.[14]

A worrying dimension that was apparent in the questionnaire comments in 2007 was the association in a student's view between being black and 'doing the dirty work'. This insight came from a comment made by a first year student who saw 'race' rather than stage of training or student status as a reason for being expected to do the 'dirty work' by the ward hierarchy (both HCAs and staff nurse).

She said:

> I was used as an extra person to get the workload done by the care assistants. They had you doing all the work while they were on long breaks. And the staff nurse who did not want to clean patient faeces asked me and a third year student to clean it up even though we were busy with another patient. As we were both black, we felt used as if that's what people thought we were there for.

Lecturers and clinical staff in the qualitative component of the 2007 study (who were predominantly 'White British') described the clinical learning environment as being influenced by the multicultural nature of the student and staff population, which they perceived had led to different experiences of, and expectations towards learning. Concern was expressed that a more diverse workforce had led to different ways of learning which were not easy to accommodate in busy clinical environments. Furthermore they felt that these differences were not being addressed openly within either the NHS Trusts or the universities.

For one ward manager the difficulties were because:

A lot of our workforce haven't been educated in the same system and that is something that culturally there are differences and training wise, it's not a question of knowledge base or anything like that, but it is a system that is different and I think for a lot of the staff if they haven't experienced hierarchy in the workforce, they find it difficult if someone perceived as higher in the hierarchy like the matron knows something that you don't …. And breaking down those barriers and preconceived ideas has actually been quite difficult, to get a team that's gelled and feel that yes, you can challenge, you can approach your seniors, you can do all of those things.

Another manager said:

I think there's a huge under-estimation of differences in communication terms, everything. I think there are huge differences and it makes a hell of a difference to the care we're delivering, and I don't think people take that on board.

Similar issues were also reported in the overseas nurses' study, where it was found that managers and mentors appeared to have a limited understanding of equal opportunities and therefore failed to address the difficulties evoked through working in a multicultural workforce (Smith et al. 2006). One issue that emerged as a recurrent theme was the use of English by overseas nurses from Commonwealth countries which was regarded as 'different' and often negatively by indigenous British English speakers. Emotional labour appeared to be undertaken on the one hand to conceal negative emotions felt by the 'indigenous' workforce and by the 'overseas' nurses on the other as part of 'fitting in'.[15]

Summary

In this chapter I have described how in the 1980s nurses defined the physical, technical and emotional components of their work according to medical specialities. But students frequently found themselves in emotionally charged situations. These situations went beyond the medical and technical definitions of their training and back to nursing as people work. This was reflected in the way in which students used patients' personal characteristics as well as what was 'wrong' with them as a way of describing their work and learning. Thus patients' age, gender, racial characteristics and whether they were appreciative also shaped the way in which they saw their work.

Students frequently engaged in emotional labour in these emotionally charged situations. Often they experienced anxiety and stress because their emotional labour was neither formally recognized nor valued as part of 'real' nursing (with the possible exceptions of oncology and psychiatry) nor incorporated into the theoretical and practical organization of their training. How then did emotional labour, the invisible and undervalued component of nursing, get reproduced in the wards?

Further conclusions for the 2000s suggest that the need for reflection to manage emotions continues to go largely unmet[16] and yet is particularly pertinent given the increased complexity of the work environment in which students and others find themselves, together with the speed up and short patient stays experienced in the acute clinical context. Perhaps this lack of opportunity to reflect is indicative of a wider shift to skills and competency-based education and practice identified by Scott (2004), who describes a move away from relational caring where emotions are not identified as a key component of nursing and therefore not taught or assessed in education or practice. Findings from the 2007 study suggest that emotions remain a strong feature of learning, mentoring and practice and that support is required to focus on how to manage feelings and learn from them. Emotional labour continues to be an invisible and undervalued component of nursing in the complex settings and systems of twenty-first century health care and education, in which the students find themselves learning to be nurses. So how then does it get reproduced in the clinical context of the contemporary NHS? This question will be the subject of Chapter 5.

5

The ward sister and the infrastructure of emotion work: making it visible on the ward – from ward sister to ward manager and the role of the mentor

In the original study it was found that the ward sister created the infrastructure which allowed the production and reproduction of emotional labour in placements by setting the emotional tone through her management style. Indicators of her management style as perceived by students included: knowing the rules (i.e. that there was consistency of expectation); promoting fair and equable relationships; sharing the work; working alongside students and showing them what to do; recognizing them as a person by making them feel welcome, cared for and safe.

These findings are revisited by investigating the current clinical leadership arrangements for the organization and delivery of education to student nurses in the clinical setting particularly in relation to the role of the mentor associated with the major changes following the introduction of the Project 2000 and Fitness to Practice curricula. Parallel developments saw the erosion of the traditional ward sister's role, which was replaced by the ward manager. How then has the relationship between the good nurse and the good ward sister in the production and reproduction of emotional labour in the clinical setting as portrayed in the first book been transformed into the nurse manager's and mentor's roles; and what effects does this transformation have on student nurses and patients?

In the first book I claimed that 'In the "real world" of the ward, emotion work was neither formally recognized nor valued as part of nursing. But nurses still engaged in it'.

After 20 years the ward is still regarded as the 'real world', not the university where most of the student's formal learning takes place. Although committed to caring, students now talk of a distinctive hierarchy of nursing skills, differentiated by personal care delivered by health care assistants (HCAs) and technical skills undertaken by registered nurses to whom they are aspiring rather than by stage of training.

Everybody's ideal: characteristics of ward sisters and nurses

In the mid-1980s, I asked what were the conditions that permitted the production and reproduction of emotional labour? My research suggested at that time that the answer lay with the ward sister, who, as the architect of nursing work and organization, was seen to set the emotional agenda (i.e. the feeling rules) of the ward. The ward sister was clearly recognized as a type and a product of the specific cultural environment of the City hospital. She was described as everyone's ideal who not only 'looked like a model' but was calm, kind, considerate and 'got the work done on time'. When the nurses felt appreciated and supported emotionally by the ward sisters, they not only had a role model for emotionally explicit patient care, but they also felt able to care for patients in this way.

The characteristics of the 'ideal' nurse, frequently modelled on a much admired ward sister, were interchangeable and represented the high expectations nurses had for themselves and each other, and which were passed on from one generation to the next.

Technical competency and specialist knowledge alone did not dominate the picture, as the importance of the emotional component of caring as an explicit management style began to emerge. This finding was substantiated by data from interviews with ward sisters with at least 20 years' nursing experience in which they described the constancy of the characteristics of the 'ideal' nurse, passed on from one generation of nurses to the next and their admiration of and aspiration to achieve both technical competency and emotional literacy. Characteristics included: 'a very good organiser, a very good practical nurse and she really cared for the well-being of the patients. She really cared for them as a person'; '(She was) competent and caring. She had very good practical skills, but she would do the little things for patients and leave them feeling very much better'. Another role model demonstrated 'hard work, high standards and personal involvement with staff and patients'.

Involvement rather than hierarchy was seen to be paramount in order to counter a system 'where the sister made people so nervous that you were actually afraid to express how you felt about anything and you couldn't develop your own role because you were suppressed by her system'. Knowing the rules was another consistent theme. Students liked to know what was expected of them during a ward allocation as these two students illustrate below;

> Sister on this specialist surgical ward was very good. She sat me down on my first shift and said 'This is what I expect from a third year', so I knew where I stood from the beginning. I said to her 'If every sister did that, the wards would run so much smoother'.
>
> I think the whole [medical] ward was run very smoothly because you knew where you were. She [Sister] had rules. She let you know what the rules were.

Consistency of rules and expectations on the sister's part was one of the ways in which she created a supportive and relaxed ward atmosphere and a third-year student told me how, on her most recent allocation to an oncology ward, 'it was very easy to feel at ease on this ward' which she described as 'very good for nursing care, if you feel relaxed with *people*'. Another student described in more detail how the sister made people 'feel at ease' and 'relaxed'. 'We had a very easy-going relationship. Everybody was called by their first names and you had a real laugh'.

In the current climate of the 2010s this consistency was not so easy to identify. Despite the mentor being indicated as the key person with whom the student related to in terms of their learning, the reality was very variable and they could be exposed to a variety of other qualified nurses throughout their placements. This student's experience was not uncommon. She said:

> I haven't spent very much time with my mentor or associate mentor so I've just been allocated with various nurses depending on who's on and who I've worked with the previous day.

In the 1980s, there had been a more consistently clear connection in the students' minds between their own positive learning experiences' and the ward sisters' approach to patients and their relatives. The students clearly admired those ward sisters who took their time to talk to patients and their relatives, staying overtime to do this 'if someone is upset'. This behaviour signified to students that 'sister is genuinely concerned about the patients', which motivated them to 'really want to do things for people on that ward'.

The sister's ability to create good social relations among nursing staff was a critical component of the ward atmosphere as indicated in the following student comments:

> Sisters are critical because of their influence on staff nurses. They in turn influence how the students work and on the way they feel, their morale.

Sister's attitude is very important. On sister depends the happiness of staff nurses and students.

The significance of creating good social relations between the nurses on the ward becomes evident when we consider the hierarchical nature of nursing. We can draw on the example given by the ward sister above to illustrate the potential use of this 'hierarchy system' to make subordinates feel nervous, afraid, suppressed. A student gives similar insights who described the ward sister as 'undoubtedly critical ... undoubtedly the key .... She sets the pace'.

A student who had just finished on a ward described the effects of an authoritarian management style which produced anxiety in the staff nurses 'because they felt responsible to sister' with the result 'they had to "check" the students 'every inch of the way'.

Students were also very critical of ward sisters, and sometimes their staff nurses, who sat in their offices behind closed doors 'sending the orders down'. The physical separation of the trained staff from the students reinforced the hierarchical nature of the social relations between them, and as one student observed 'the trained staff never really get to know us as people. On the last ward you weren't allowed in the office if anybody trained was there. We'd have to go in the day room with the patients'.

On the other hand, a student thought that:

Students work jolly hard if they are working with somebody who understands them a bit more and thanks them at the end of the shift, rather than bossing them around all the time.

Thus the mark of the good ward sister was the one who was out there on the ward caring for patients alongside students. Through her contact with patients she 'kept in touch' and was able 'to see the amount of work students do'. As another student said:

When they're out there on the ward you feel you can go and talk to them. They're much more approachable than when they're sitting in their little office.

The ideal sister did not supervise in the way of the sister who created anxiety for her staff and students by checking 'every inch of the way'. Rather she took an 'interest in what you are doing and how you are *feeling* about the ward. She makes sure the work is allocated fairly and within the students' capabilities. She also says "I'll come and help you" if you haven't done it before'.

A tutor summed up the characteristics of the 'ideal ward environment' created by the sister, confirming the students' views described above. She said:

The ideal environment is where there is consistency, teamwork and where you don't have a hierarchical 'us and them' situation. The students see fairness and consistency because the sister and staff nurses roll up their sleeves and work.

Another tutor described similar characteristics based on two actual (surgical) ward sisters working at City at that time.

> These two sisters create an efficient and effective environment and they are regarded with affection by the nurses. The atmosphere on their wards is very safe. They are extremely approachable and very clear-cut in what they want and the students know exactly where they are with them.

The hierarchical ward sister also created feeling rules based on hierarchy, authority and often unattainable high standards of patient care which prioritized technical competency and efficiency at the expense of their own, their juniors' and patients' emotional needs. Students and staff nurses on these wards were likely to experience negative feelings (fear, anxiety and suppression of their own feelings) as a consequence of the sister's hierarchical management style.

One student summed it up:

> Fear isn't a good way to learn to care. Mutual respect is the best. If you feel appreciated you try to live up to the faith people have in you. It's a very strong stimulus.

The view was consistently expressed that patients, like nurses, were sensitive to ward atmospheres created by the sister (as Revans had reported in 1964). Patients knew if the students were not happy or if the morale was low.

Producing and reproducing emotional labour in the ward

When I undertook my study in the 1980s, the sisters managed their wards to set the emotional tone to make the students, and hence the patients, feel safe and cared for in a convivial environment as opposed to frightened, anxious and defensive? In what ways did they make these feeling rules explicit?

In the 1980s, staff nurses at the City Hospital chose to work on particular wards because they had usually worked there as students based on their positive experiences of both the speciality and the sister's particular management style. One sister confirmed this view explaining that the staff nurses 'recruit themselves really. They work on the wards as students, the majority of them, and then if they enjoyed the ward they ask if they can come back for consolidation and if there's a vacancy and if they're interested and they're satisfactory at interview, they're appointed'.

But the implication of what the sister is saying is that she recruited staff nurses who would reproduce an explicitly emotional caring style. Thus, the sisters and staff nurses not only chose to work together because they liked each other's philosophy and style, but developed into a cohesive group over a period of at least a year. Students and patients, on the other hand, stayed for much shorter periods on the wards and did not usually have much say over their placements or admissions. In 2007, students' future career choices were more likely to be determined by market forces i.e. where the jobs were available although their final three-month placement at the end of their third year was designed to allow them to select an area on the basis of preferences built up during their training.

In the climate of the 1980s sisters were crucial in setting the emotional tone or feeling rules of the ward, and it is likely that their work preferences and priorities were determined by their own particular rationality of care rather than the medical speciality of the ward. Furthermore, nurses at City had some sense of the nursing process as a patient-orientated rather than task-orientated work method. Although on all the wards I worked one or two nurses were assigned on each shift to look after a group of patients (average of six per shift), most sisters still operated a system that enabled them to supervise and control the students (Davies 1976). Even when they allocated the work by patients, the sisters made it clear there were certain tasks and routines that had to be completed by a set time.

I used Davies' (1990) mode of analysis to look at patient-centred tasks and routines, shaped by medical diagnosis and treatment (doctors' rounds and varieties of diagnostic tests and therapies on and off the ward), which she described as the 'assembly line [rather than the nurturing] care of the sick'. On some wards, sisters as well as doctors were motivated by medical diagnosis and treatment rather than a nurturing approach which led them to organize the nursing work in this way.

A third-year student was critical of the emphasis on routines, believing that it prevented students from questioning their care. She said: 'On some wards the care is just too routinised. You just do things and you don't question'.

A student, only weeks into her training, motivated to care for people rather than diseases, soon realized that the running of a hospital was in opposition to the people-centred ethos of the nursing process and a more nurturing approach to patient care. She said:

> I mean hospitals aren't run for the individual patient, they're run for everybody, aren't they? It would be nice if they could be geared to each person but they can't really, can they?

Her question is a pertinent one for both the 1980s and the current target-driven context of the NHS. This question of institutionally versus individually driven care was at the centre of a number of classic research studies cited by Evers (1984), which influenced my analysis in the first study i.e. how possible is it to meet individual needs within an institution? King and colleagues (1971) used Goffman's typology of total institutions (1968) for measuring the degree of client-centredness within childcare institutions. Miller and Gwynne (1972) discovered that chronically disabled residents in long-stay institutions were either encouraged as individuals (the horticultural model of care) or were the recipients of impersonal routines (the warehousing model of care). Evers (1984) applied their analysis to the care of the elderly in the wards of a geriatric hospital. She found that the different orientations on a ward towards either the horticultural or the warehousing model was primarily dependent on the ward sister's leadership and priorities.[1]

These findings showed that client or institutional orientation on a ward or unit depended on the attitudes of the supervisor or sister. Similar findings emerged from my own study, focusing particularly on how the sister set the emotional tone of the ward. It was this emotional tone and how she set it (her emotional management style) that in part answered the student's question as to how possible it was to gear the needs of the institution to 'each person'. I found that when a ward sister had an express commitment to the nursing process person-centred philosophy, she was more likely to use it as a work method to create the infrastructure which allowed the production and reproduction of emotional labour in her ward. How did she do this?

Reproducing emotional labour, management styles and the nursing process

In the 1980s, the sisters on the wards I observed were all committed to the person-orientated approach of the nursing process, but they interpreted its work method in different ways. They were all patient-centred to varying degrees, but the amount of contact they had with doctors varied according to speciality. In the more specialized wards, where patients were undergoing a battery of medical tests and investigations, the sisters and doctors worked more closely together. On the general medical wards, more patients were well advanced in their illness trajectory. Often they were entering a chronic phase and tended to be more dependent on nursing care than medical intervention. Here, the sisters and doctors had less contact with each other. Whatever the case, the sisters did not lose sight of either the patients or the students, but some clearly saw patient care as their top priority while others saw teaching students as an integral part of that priority. The sister on Edale ward said: 'I see that it's my responsibility to ensure the patients get good care and one of the ways to ensure this is to teach the students how'. The sister's commitment to teaching was reflected in high scores on the learning environment questionnaire (see: Companion website, Appendix E, Tables E8, E9 and E10, Smith 1992).

Similarly in 2007, as described in Chapter 4, positive associations were found between quality of care, satisfaction with placements and a perception that trained staff worked with learners. The decrease in the mean scores (out of 5.0) for ward/placement teaching from 3.46 in 1984 to 3.12 in 2007 suggested that the gap is perceived to be even wider between students' expectations for formal teaching in placements and what qualified staff actually provided. Other changes that could explain the decrease may be attributed to the transformation of the ward sister's role into a variety of manager and specialist roles and responsibilities of which student learning was just one component. On the other hand the increase in the students' mean ratings of their perceived learning opportunities from 2.76 in 1984 to 3.56 in 2007 may indicate that their supernumerary status as learners rather than workers had raised awareness of their need to learn while on practice placements (see: Companion website, Methodological Appendix II, Smith 2012).

Turning specifically to the role of emotion work in student learning, I was interested to find in 1984 that it was not officially legitimized by the medical speciality of each of the four wards where I undertook participant observation. Even though a number of patients on all the wards were suffering from cancer, because none of them were officially oncology wards, death and dying were not on the medically legitimized agenda.

On Ronda ward, many of the patients were suffering from a variety of chronic illnesses, ranging from respiratory to Alzheimer's disease, and although many of the patients were elderly, the physicians still worked in an interventionist and curative way. But the sister was more orientated towards emotion work compared with many of her colleagues.

Another student told me how she had gone 'overboard' for Ronda ward and its elderly patient population:

> My set [classmates] thought I was mad because the ward has this reputation of being just basic nursing. But Sister Ronda made me realize what an art it is to care for people who can't do very much for themselves and who rely on good personal relationships.

Yet another student who described the mechanisms used on a psychiatric ward to focus on the emotional aspects of work told me that very few general ward sisters worked in this way. She mentioned two sisters, one of whom was Sister Ronda, the other a ward sister on a care of the elderly ward who did. When I asked her why she thought they were able to work in this way, she said:

> They are both open to change. On most general wards you are expected to support a patient in depression but you're not supported yourself. You are expected to treat the patients psychologically, but nobody tells you how to do that. But these two sisters do. They are very open to change with regard to the nursing process and they try desperately hard each shift to do what is right.

During the subsequent weeks of fieldwork, I noticed that Sister Ronda spent considerable proportions of her time talking to patients, and she was the only person who clearly articulated the importance of patients' emotional support to nurses. I remember being momentarily taken by surprise when one of Ronda ward's regular patients was re-admitted. She and the sister greeted each other warmly, each giving the other a hug. I reflected on the incident for some time and then began to understand why it had made an impression on me. It was because I still expected nurses, especially ward sisters, to be distant and cool from their patients, applying their 'no touch' aseptic techniques to their personal relationships.

But this was not Sister Ronda's way. She was clearly motivated by a nurturing rationality that put people at the centre of care rather than sticking to rigid time-tables and routines. As one student put it:

> Sister Ronda doesn't mind how long it takes, but other sisters want you to get on with their routines.

Patients, as well as students, often marginalized 'talking' with nurses as an extra. I experienced this early on in the fieldwork when I was sitting, talking to a patient about her illness and treatment. At one point in the discussion she suddenly interjected: 'Oh I'm sorry I'd better not keep you from your work'. When I explained that our discussion was part of my work, she relaxed and carried on talking.

However, the situation also occurred where the physical labour could be so demanding that emotional labour took second priority. One patient told me, how when the staffing levels were low, nurses would be so rushed that even though they began conversations they might be called away before they had time to finish them.

These descriptions of time and the workload have resonances with the notion of work being constrained by a predetermined time allowance or timetable associated with a male concept of time. Students found themselves caught between the competing rationalities, not only of hospital administrators and doctors, but also their ward sisters. In the mid-1980s, Sister Ronda's obvious concern for people and recognition of communication and the development of good personal relations as part of the work were seen by many students as 'atypical' but also mildly eccentric and at times impractical. Furthermore, her emphasis on people rather than tasks could be seen as changing a system which, as Menzies (1960) suggested, served as a defence against student anxiety.

In what ways then did Sister Ronda organize and manage nursing in a way that made her management style emotionally different to many of her colleagues? First of all, it was the way in which she allocated and distributed the work based on individual nurses caring for specific patients. Many of the students, used to the more usual practice on other wards of patient-centred tasks found Sister Ronda's emphasis on patient-centred care difficult to deal with. Their reaction was part of feeling that organizing care in a patient-centred way took more time than was available, because it also meant 'getting to know them', especially for patients who had a high level of physical dependency. Getting to know patients and being in continuous contact with them also meant that nurses were required to manage their feelings more than when they operated at the level of getting through tasks.

Personal relationships were at the centre of Sister Ronda's interactions, and emotional needs were openly identified and articulated. The students' top questionnaire ratings of Ronda ward's positive ward atmosphere/staff relations were evidence of this. (see: Companion website, Appendix E, Table E11, Smith 1992).

Another student, speaking for many, was reluctant to look after patients on a continuous basis during their hospital stay. One reason for her reluctance seemed to be associated with the increased demand for emotional labour. She said:

> It depends really on striking the balance between getting to know the patients well and knowing what's going on in the rest of the ward. And not letting say a certain patient getting to the point of irritating you.

On the majority of the wards the trained staff held the view that students should be given some choice over who they looked after and for how long. As one student explained (and which I saw verified time and time again during the report), the trained staff would say:

> Who looked after so and so today? And they would then let another nurse look after him or her who hadn't looked after them for a week. I think you've got to do it like that or else the patients might become too dependent on you or you might not get on so well. I think it's just more positive for the patient to be able to change regularly.

The joy of getting through the work as a series of tasks is clearly demonstrated by the following student account:

> We worked down one end and everybody was bathed, everybody had their hair washed who wanted to and the ward was absolutely spotless. We were actually getting them bathed without them being told: 'Oh yes you can have a bath; do you really want a bath? Could you have a bath this evening?' and nobody gets a bath in the evening. It's ridiculous. We really felt we had achieved something. The patients were happy and we were happy.

This student was working on Ronda ward at the time and took the opportunity of the sister's day off to organize the work in such a way that she felt she had something to show for her physical rather than emotional labours. Putting patients at the centre of their care was seen by her as time consuming (and anxiety provoking?), and she believed that everyone was happy partly because the patients had not had to make their own choices but had been fitted into routines.

In the case of Sister Ronda she used handovers and reports for discussing with each individual nurse the proposed care for the day and then evaluated it with them at the end of the shift. The language used during the handovers on Ronda ward was often very different to that used on the more technically orientated wards.

One student captured the spirit of the ward handovers on Ronda ward when she said:

> Sister always stressed talking and it was the things you said rather than what you did ... like she actually wanted you to describe the content of the conversations you'd had with patients. You couldn't just say words like 'encourage' or 'reassure'. You actually had to say what you'd done to encourage or reassure someone.

By way of contrast, on Edale ward, a technically orientated ward with an emphasis on patients' vital signs, fluid balance and preparation for medical investigations, a student experienced the ward reports in the following way:

> You're not expected to know about people how they feel. I found it difficult in report sometimes. The trained staff would be saying things that I knew about because I'd talked to the patients about them. But they didn't want to know.

To sum up, on Ronda ward the sister's emotional management style was such that both patients and nurses felt valued by her, and as one student said:

> Sister really cares I'm sure. She really does seem to care, so I do too.

My 1980s case study data allowed me to examine the infrastructure of emotion work on the ward, which led me to conclude that the emotional tone was set by the ward sister in a variety of ways. Efficiency and competence were essential but were further enhanced by the ward sister's positive emotional style. I also found that ward sisters' and students' ideal nurses shared a number of key characteristics. Experienced sisters and the students valued a nurse with a 'caring' side and who was people-orientated. The nursing process could then be regarded as a way of formalizing the nurse's traditional caring role. Favourable management styles were demonstrated by sisters who were happy, approachable, accessible, valued talking and communication and gave positive feedback.

When the nurses felt appreciated and supported emotionally by the sisters, they not only had a role model for emotionally explicit patient care, but they also felt better able to care for patients in this way. Patients and nurses were sensitive to the ward atmosphere and social relations created by the sister. The assumption is that technical and physical labours are enhanced when underpinned by an emotionally explicit caring style. It was the ward sister's emotional management style that in part answered the student's question as to how possible it was to gear the needs of the institution to 'each person'. The nursing process philosophy and work method created greater emotional involvement for students (which the task allocation method helped them to avoid) and could potentially increase their anxiety. Overall, however, I found that when a ward sister had an express commitment to the nursing process person-centred philosophy, she was more likely to use it as a work method to create the infrastructure which allowed the production and reproduction of emotional labour in her ward.

The ward learning environment in 2006–2008

Managers and mentors

In recent fieldwork the ward sister was no longer clearly identified or visible in the way s/he had been in the 1980s. Given the ensuing changes within the NHS during the 1990s and 2000s the ward sister's role and indeed that of the staff nurse was reconfigured into a series of clinical and educational roles at different grades and levels of experience led by a senior nurse usually designated as a ward manager. This ward manager was supported by an increasing number of senior nurses in diverse roles such as modern matrons, practice development nurses, specialist nurses such as pain nurses, tissue viability nurses, diabetes nurses to name but a few. In terms of the new educational roles these included link lecturers, practice educators (PEs), clinical placement facilitators who contributed to supporting the student's clinical learning through the mentor either directly or indirectly. As Magnusson and colleagues observe: 'The individual role descriptions differ and indeed also their titles, but they all have the common aim of improving and strengthening practice learning for healthcare students through supporting students, mentors and practice staff' (2007, p .644).

During fieldwork for example, I noted that on any one shift there could be a variety of qualified nurses on duty who described themselves as staff nurses, ward sisters and the ward manager. A variety of grades, competences and roles were attached to these designations;[2] being a mentor was one of them. When asked who their mentors were students gave a very mixed picture, describing them as senior staff nurses, staff nurses and sometimes a ward sister or ward manager. The ideal mentor was 'a dead good nurse' and very experienced and approachable. Students also mentioned that sometimes the mentor may have only recently qualified, but this meant they were still relatively close to the student experience which made them more accessible and understanding. Some students described the ward manager or ward sister as taking on the associate mentor role 'so they're there as back up for you'. Students usually preferred the ward manager or ward sister to be associate mentors because 'they run the ward and have to do the administration whereas if the staff nurse is your mentor they spend most of their time on the ward so that you can actually get to work with them'.

But for one student, having the ward manager as a mentor had been 'brilliant' because:

> Everyone respected her. She was quite strict but you got the job done, so it made me remember more. She let me do quite a lot and I was taking my own patients and thinking for myself as well. But because she was quite strict it made me think 'oh I've got to do it!'

So like the ward sisters in the previous study there was a sense that students learnt if there were clear expectations for their learning by the ward leader.

Ward learning demanded give and take on the part of the mentor but also the student. A mentor who was an experienced staff nurse described her role as promoting 'an atmosphere in which people feel happy learning in' while students agreed that:

> If you've got a good mentor you learn so much more but you get out of it what you put in and you have to get what you need out of that placement.

Good communication skills on both sides were also seen as essential. One student said:

> If you communicate well with your mentor they'll communicate well with you.

One student described how:

> If you show to them that you're willing and you're keen and you want to learn and you're there because you want to learn, then you will get that back.

Another student was very conscious that:

> There are times when you're with your mentor and you're looking after this patient but there might be a time when your mentor at that moment in time has just got to get this situation under control and as a student you take a step back and you let them have that space.

A student who had the ward manager as her mentor thought that:

> Because I was a third year and nearing the end of my training, and because obviously the ward manager has got so much to do I think it helped her when she was on the ward because I was working with her, so I took some of her workload off her.

The ability to be aware of the mentor's needs was particularly apparent in 'mature' students. One mature student said:

> I mean how many times have you been older than your mentor? I have, lots of times and I think just from my experiences, my age, my maturity, I can gauge when she's had enough and you just need to back off a bit.

Another student commented that:

Some students think that the ward revolves around them and it doesn't, it revolves around the patients and some students get very upset if they don't actually work with their mentors, but obviously to me that's immaturity – you have to go out there and get what you want from the placement. But you know it's about being flexible.

Her colleague responded:

Yeah. I've said it a few times to some of the younger students, if you take some of the routine tasks off your mentor, like the blood pressures, that gives them a bit of time for you so it is swings and roundabouts you know, you get what you put in.

When I asked an experienced PE and former ward sister 'who is it that student nurses learn from now?' she replied:

Well, I don't think it's any one person. It's certainly not the ward sister anymore because their role has changed so much; I would say it's their mentors. When you talk to students and if they've had a very good mentor on a ward, that seems to swing it for them. Having said that, if it's a very well run ward and they feel that they're supported and people are interested in them, even if they can't always work with their mentor because of sickness or night duty or something, they feel okay. But it's their mentors who have the biggest influence really.

The PE added:

I spoke to one student on the corridor the other day who actually stopped me to make a point of telling me how wonderful this mentor had been, and it's very often about, the student that's not very confident, it's about letting them do things and supervising them and having that specialist experience to know what they can do, because if you don't know your own specialty well how can you decide what a student can do, so this student spoke at length about this mentor who had let her do a lot of things that had made her feel more confident and it was like a sort of turning point in her career really the effect that this mentor had had on her because every day there was this kind of working together, this sort of 'right, what are we doing together', it was a partnership. So it's a lot about letting them do things, encouraging them and giving them confidence.

The point the PE makes about the knowledge of a speciality that the mentor had in order to be able to more effectively mentor the student is an interesting one, since the development of specialist nursing roles had been another change I observed since the original research. The creation of posts such as nurse consultants and specialist nurses meant that there was now another route for nurses with specialist skills, expertise and experience to pursue their careers than to become a ward-based manager with specialist expertise. This change was seen to potentially diminish the ward sister role[3] at the same time as be a loss to clinical learning as explained by one senior nurse who said:

> You've got excellent staff nurses who mentor and then become the excellent clinical nurse specialist who aren't on the wards anymore! (*Laughs*)

One participant went so far as to suggest that:

> If those specialist roles weren't there those nurses would be in the wards giving care and teaching and supporting....

Students were most likely to see nurses in these specialist roles during their 'hub and spokes'[4] practice experiences, and their mentors were described as playing a significant role in helping them to make sense of these experiences. Furthermore the role of the specialist nurses in teaching students varied. During interview with a second year student nurse about the role played by mentors and specialist nurses in her learning, she identified a team of wound care specialist nurses as people who 'really encapsulate nursing'. She said:

> I think wound care is quite essential. I've spent some time with a really good tissue viability nurse who was great at what she did and was lovely; and I think wound care is essential because it can all be about prevention as well, you know, like good nutrition and pressure sores.

In contrast, PEs were aware that many specialist nurses chose not to teach student nurses because 'they think their speciality is so specialist and at too high a level to meet the students' learning needs'. They also suggested that 'deskilling' was one of the consequences of developing specialist nursing roles distinct from the generic nursing workforce as exemplified by the development of the discharge coordinator who liaised with social and community services to prepare patients for discharge, thus denying nurse managers and nurses in general and students in particular the direct experience of making arrangements for patients to go home.

When I looked at students' perceptions of the professional groups who were most likely to teach them as expressed in their questionnaire ratings, they tended to agree that trained nurses taught them during their placements and identified them more specifically as their mentors, community and hospital specialists, ward managers and modern matrons across a range of mean scores in descending order from higher (3.78) to lower scores (2.19) (see: Companion website, Methodological Appendix II, Smith 2012).

The mentor's role has been described at some length in Chapter 2 and 3 and their importance to clinical learning highlighted. The mentor holds a pivotal position in relation to the student, their university lecturers, the clinical staff, other clinically based educators and the patient. It was also clear that the mentor could make both a positive and negative difference to the student's learning experience.

Following interviews with second and third-year students, I clustered the qualities most valued by students as follows:

- An understanding of what the student is going through
- A willingness to teach
- Knowing the student
- Telling them what to do while letting them do things by themselves
- Appreciating the students (through value, trust and respect)
- Confidence in themselves
- Experienced nurses
- Nice people
- Ability to communicate

Students were looking for:

A good general nurse, with a lot of experience at nursing who's maybe been on different wards, seen a lot of different things, a nursing sister. They'd be ideal, who have good communication skills, who are in tune with everything.

Or someone who was:

Actually interested in developing you as a nurse, especially your clinical skills

I also asked students how from their experience they thought mentors were able to best support them. Again I was able to cluster their responses into the following themes:

How mentors are best able to support students

- Building rapport, trust and relationships
- Meeting the students' learning needs
- Knowing how to look after them
- Interested in developing the student as a nurse especially clinical skills
- Being there
- Being available
- Empathy for the student
- Being friendly
- Showing encouragement
- Listening to you
- Being part of a team
- Enabling students to contribute to the workload
- Enabling the student to learn by providing the structure for learning
- Two way process: what students put in to support the mentor

Students elaborated further:

I think friendliness is a really good factor. Being able to talk to them, build a rapport with them and build a relationship as well.

One student described how her mentor:

Right from the start, completely listened to everything that I wanted to do, suggested things that would be beneficial to me and took the time out, if I didn't understand something, to actually sit down with me and go through it, and she actually arranged when we were working nights and it wasn't particularly busy, she actually spent the time to do some teaching sessions with me. Another thing, they've made me feel like it's a safe environment to actually have a go and build my confidence.

Another student mentioned the ward ethos as important where enthusiasm and motivation and a 'humanistic approach' made students feel welcome.

My findings suggest that mentors now set the emotional tone of the students' learning. Occasionally the ward manager could also be a student mentor but was more likely to be their associate. Students recognized that the ward managers had other responsibilities which took them away from their mentoring commitments and therefore on balance preferred their mentors to be senior staff nurses. Good relationships and rapport articulated through the mentor make the students feel welcome, safe and part of the ward team. Positive relationships, rapport and team working continue to be set by the emotional tone of the former ward sister (now manager) and are essential to the students' emotional wellbeing, safety and learning. The students' insights are also confirmed by the views of an experienced PE and former ward sister. We now explore these issues in greater depth below.

From ward sister to ward manager: who sets the emotional tone?

In relation to the role of the ward sister as conceived in the 1980s as a specialist-based practitioner this role had transformed into that of ward manager who manages and interacts with a range of clinical nurse specialists and educationalists. Changes in ward leadership and workforce organization since the completion of the first study meant that supervision of direct patient care and student learning were delegated by ward managers to other qualified staff. When I requested information about a patient or student from the ward manager whom I perceived to be the person in charge, I was invariably told to speak to the member of staff who had been 'looking after' either the patient or student for that shift because they would have the in-depth knowledge readily available.

Given my original premise on the key role of the ward sister, the question became urgent as to whom the students identified with as their role models, and who set the emotional tone to ensure the production and reproduction of emotional labour from one generation of nurses to the next. Overall, however the ward manager was seen to play a key leadership role for student nurse learning, albeit in a different way to her ward sister predecessor and supported by nurses in new clinical and educational roles, although occasionally the ward manager could also be a student mentor.

Five PEs who had worked as traditional ward sisters were now supporting the creation of the ward learning environment for student nurses but in a different way. As one educator observed, the ward manager led student nurse learning by creating the necessary conditions 'behind the scenes' to ensure the smooth running of the ward to provide the necessary backdrop for learning to take place. She said:

How a ward is run has a bearing overall. If it is not well run and disorganized, it is difficult for them (the students). A well-run ward makes the students feel supported in general.

And another PE added:

I think the Ward Manager has an impact 'full stop.' If the ward's well run and organized, educational learning is more easily facilitated. You see I'm very lucky because I've got a fantastic Ward Manager and it's a nice area to work in, so learning's easy.

Thus in these PEs' eyes the ward manager was seen to lead ward learning 'at a distance' by working with and delegating to others with explicit responsibilities for student learning such as the PEs and mentors. During focus group discussion one PE described how her ward manager enabled her to successfully undertake her role:

It's the support that you get as well that influences the education that you're able to give. I have a very supportive manager and it makes a big difference to me…I mean, my Ward Manager doesn't have any input really, in all honesty, in education whatsoever, but is very supportive in anything that other people want to do. So in that aspect, she allows education to take place, but she actually has no input whatsoever into it.

Another PE, based on her own experiences added:

My Ward Manager is very good at management without you realizing. You have no idea what she's doing until it's done and you don't even resent her when you realize. She's never confrontational, unless she has to be, unless there's a real problem and even then, when she tells you off, she's very nice. If you go to her with a problem, she makes you talk it through and you'll answer your own question, so she's never really telling you what to do, you're telling yourself.

From the educator's account it appears that the ward manager undertakes emotional labour at a distance to create a 'calm working environment', which at the same time serves as a buffer which protects her staff. As a consequence the PE felt safe and cared for which in turn empowered her to make decisions.

She added:

> I think one of my Ward Manager's big, positive points is she knows who she delegates to. She does delegate, but she always delegates to the right person to do the right job. She keeps a tight control in that you always have to feed back to her, but she delegates well.

This ward manager's emotional labour extended to knowing how to delegate to the right person for the job, monitoring it and establishing a feedback loop.

In the 2007 survey I wanted to look at the associations between ward teaching and learning and the promotion of positive ward atmosphere and staff relations. Single items were selected to demonstrate students' perceptions of teaching and learning, team work and the provision of a positive ward atmosphere during their most recent placement.

The four most highly rated items out of 43 were: 'I am happy with the experience I have had on this placement'; 'there is much to learn on this placement'; 'sister and trained staff work as a team with learners'; 'sister and trained staff provide an atmosphere which is good to work in' and were indicative of the emotional labour undertaken by the ward manager/sister and her team in relation to how they set the emotional tone to support students and their learning.

When the ratings on all seven items on the ward atmosphere/staff relations dimension were combined to obtain a mean score of 3.62 out of 5.0 for all placements, it compared favorably with the 1984 score of 3.77 for 12 wards, suggesting that ward atmosphere/staff relations continue to play a major role in promoting the wellbeing of staff, students which in turn influences their learning (see: Chapter 4 and Companion website, Methodological Appendix II, Smith 2012).

The changing infrastructure of emotional labour and learning in the 2000s

From fieldwork observations, practitioners and students' accounts, it appeared that the structure of the learning environment was more diverse than it had been at the time of the first study in general and in the City Hospital environment in particular. Added to this was the change in the structure of the nursing workforce and the fragmentation of the leadership for learning and caring.

The ward handovers, written and verbal reports, were also measures of the ward sister's management style and the orientation which underpinned it. Senior nurses who had been at the frontline of clinical care since the 1980s recalled that students used to be encouraged to ask questions during ward handovers but that this was no longer the case from a workforce who felt being under pressure and therefore less amenable to putting themselves into situations where their knowledge could be challenged.

Observation of and participation in handovers in the 2000s showed that they had become much more focused and target driven than in the 1980s when the handovers were far more discursive and used for teaching as well as communication purposes. Now the main aim of the ward handover was to exchange sufficient information between shifts in the minimum time possible in order to ensure the effective and efficient delivery of patient care and not primarily as 'an occasion for teaching learners' as reflected in student responses to the questionnaire statement 'The shift handover is used as an occasion for teaching learners' in which a low mean score of 2.72 out of 5.0 was obtained.

PEs also reported that they rather than the ward managers took on 'a trouble-shooting role' to ensure the student's successful completion of a placement which might require complex negotiation with key stakeholders (including as well as on behalf of the ward manager) across a range of issues (e.g. supporting mentors, monitoring students' paperwork, dealing with underachieving or 'failing' students). The success of such complex negotiations relied on the PEs establishing a good relationship with the ward managers and mentors but also on the ward managers knowing how best to work with them.

In another focus group, a discourse emerged in which managers, ward sisters and PEs described how ward managers *used* to work with students but that the role had become 'very busy' resulting in the need to develop an arms' length relationship with student learning. This discourse was confirmed during observations of ward sisters at work on a variety of medical and surgical wards. Some of them delivered care, all coordinated medical and nursing staff and managed discharges, but none of them in this group said they worked directly with students.

The following extract from my co-researcher's field notes illustrates the sister's changed role:

> Sister said her role had changed lately – whereas 10 years ago she'd taken patients and not coordinated the ward, now she coordinated the ward rather than taking patients. Therefore she doesn't work with students but 'keeps an eye'. She feels she has overall responsibility for students and supports mentors.

One PE explained to me why mentors required support and resources from the ward manager:

> Mentors are expected to care for patients at the same time as teaching students which can put them under a lot of pressure. In ICU for example, they could be caring for a very sick patient and at the same time having to orientate a new student.

Thus as these findings show, clinical learning continues to be part of the ward manager's remit and although they are supported by PEs, mentors, ward sisters,

staff nurses, clinical nurse specialists and modern matrons they hold the overall responsibility for ensuring that the learning environment, including mentor
training and support, is provided at ward level. However, due to an increased
workload, including Trust-wide responsibilities, their presence and attention have
been taken away from students and patients in many ways.

In particular, the ward managers reported that their role had been affected by
the target-driven nature of the NHS in general and acute NHS Trusts in particular. This view is apparent in the following quote. The narrator was a lead nurse
who had worked as a ward sister during the 1980s. When asked how the ward
manager's role had changed over 20 years she made the following comments:

> Obviously the NHS climate has changed. I think the target culture is here and is
> unavoidable. Obviously financial things, I have been much more aware. When I was a
> ward sister, while I had a budget for the ward, it wasn't a priority and our management
> accountant sent us messages every now and then if we were running into trouble.

Other ward managers confirmed that their role had changed fairly recently, following the introduction of targets brought in to maintain bed occupancy and throughput in a commission led NHS (Department of Health 2004c). It appeared that these
changes had impacted on ward managers by requiring them to become more outward looking and externally focused than in the previous 20 years as suggested by
the following exchange between the researcher (R) and the ward manager (WM):

> R: One of the key roles that we're hypothesising has changed has been the ward
> manager role. Do you think it's changed since you've been doing it?
>
> WM: The ward manager role? Out of all recognition! [*Laughs*] I've been a ward
> sister in different guises since the early 80s and initially it was patient focused and
> training staff and student focused and that's where your work lay but now although I
> do have a reputation for running the ward a bit like that, you are being dragged into
> all sorts of political things.

These 'political things' included an increased involvement in activities outside
the ward involving the implementation of NHS policies to meet financial and
clinical targets.

For example, in an interview with a ward manager, it became clear on further
questioning that measures 'to increase throughput in the hospital' included the
introduction of supernumerary status (i.e. no longer part of the hands on workforce) for medical ward sisters with 'frightening' effects from which she had to
'pull back':

> Yes. Well yes, supernumerary status ... we were actually doing full time, doing 5
> days a week and having to do everything within 5 days, and certainly the priority
> is to increase discharges and there's no mistake made about that, it is to increase

the through put in the hospital and you become a sort of, I don't know – what would you call it? ... You're just like an automaton, I sometimes come into the ward and I'm looking at the board as numbers (not patients) and I get quite frightened sometimes because I'm forgetting that they're people and I have to pull back.

During fieldwork it became evident that the target-driven NHS had had an impact on the way in which care was delivered in the wards, and a move away from a more holistic approach to care in the 1980s, promoted by the nursing process, to a modified form of task allocation associated with the ward staff's response to the pressure of meeting targets which required them to organize their work into a series of tasks to enable them to do so.

In the target-driven NHS the pace is busier and the patients sicker and more dependent than in the past, which means the learning is different. Task allocation in its new form is organized to meet discharge and bed targets by delivering trained nursing and HCA tasks. Consequently, a system of 'team' or 'sides' nursing (by which different groups of nurses and HCAs are allocated to work on separate 'sides' of the ward) has been introduced resulting in an apparent move away from patient-centred care.

It was also interesting to observe how ward managers allocated the work compared to in the past when in Sister Ronda's case she discussed patient allocation with the students. Now it was either a discussion related to allocation of student to mentor, or as in one student's view, a 'do it yourself' approach.

As elaborated in Chapter 7, to some extent how the work was allocated related to changes in and staff's expectations of student nurses' supernumerary status which required them to negotiate their position with their mentor and the ward team in each placement in order to be effective learners. On some wards, managers allocated the work during handovers at the beginning of the shift in order to ensure students met their learning needs:

Sister organized the work, everyone hung around the desk as she looked at the patient dependency, the staff and students. She asked students what they wanted to do, whether their mentors were on duty and knew that one third year student had a drugs assessment coming up.

In other areas, allocation of students to work with their mentors was not so well organized. A third year student said:

I wait to see – is my mentor going to sort me out? If obviously not – then I decide what I want to do and who I need to do it with.

In one Accident and Emergency (A&E) Department the consequences of this 'haphazard' approach to allocation was observed:

During handover, Sister gave out areas of A&E to different staff – then went through the six student nurses on duty – She didn't ask who had worked with their mentor, who was mentoring whom, or who needed to learn what. She then allocated students to three or four mentors randomly. The student I was working with said her mentor was working in a different area to her but she decided not to argue the need to work with her mentor during the shift even though to date she hadn't worked with him during this placement.

In this account the student had made her own decision just to get on with her allocated work and not to use her supernumerary status to negotiate with the ward manager to ensure she worked with her mentor. The effort involved in negotiating supernumerary status successfully is not to be underestimated and requires emotional labour on the part of the student to do this with ward staff who are sensitive to their needs and who make them feel welcome and part of a team.

As one student put it:

You want somebody who recognizes that you're their student and you know, like, 'you're with me' and makes you feel welcome.

Another student concluded:

The best mentor includes you in what they're doing. You have your handover and then you're put with your mentor and it's like 'Right, this is what we're going to do. You do this. I'll do that.' And then halfway through the work maybe say 'Right, let's go through what needs doing and where we are up to with the patients.' And also somebody who says 'thank you' at the end of the shift for your help. That's really nice because you feel like it's been worthwhile, what you've done.

Students also recognized that they played an active role in negotiating their supernumerary status:

It's just about becoming part of the team and saying 'yes, I am supernumerary and I am here as a student nurse but I want to contribute', and I think if you go in with that positive attitude 'I'm here and I want to contribute' then they (the mentors) will respect that and you definitely get out of it what you put in, definitely.

Summary

One of the consequences of students acquiring supernumerary status has been that they are no longer available to give 75 per cent of the direct patient care as had been the case at the time of the first study. Consequently there has been a change in skill mix, and HCAs have become prominent in the workforce of the 2000s in taking over direct patient care. Personal care is now delegated to the HCAs leaving the technical tasks to the qualified nurses. The effects on students are complex. Recent data suggest that trained nurses focus on technical tasks which only trained nurses can do, while students continue to deliver the unqualified care, which may be supervised by HCAs. This concentration and division of labour between trained and untrained workers has led to students dividing nursing work into high and low status tasks. If bedside care continues to be regarded as low status work as found by these authors and which recent data suggest continues to be the case among student nurses, then being associated with low status tasks may lead them to feeling unprepared for their future role. This is because they see themselves as undertaking low status work supervised by HCAs rather than the technical high status tasks they expect to perform on qualifying as staff nurses.

The development of a successful mentoring relationship therefore was shown to be essential to student nurse learning and dependent on the ward having a welcoming attitude to students, not seeing them as a pair of hands and offering them clear learning opportunities.

The ward manager has evolved from the ward sister role and new clinical and educational roles have developed over the intervening years to take on board different aspects of student learning (e.g. link lecturers, PEs, mentors) and patient care (e.g. modern matrons, clinical nurse specialists, nurse practitioners). However the ward manager retains overall responsibility for the emotional tone of the clinical environment within the hospital, including mentor training and support. The nursing process which was introduced during the 1970s and 1980s and gave a holistic focus to the role has now largely been abandoned due to the pressure to achieve targets. Task allocation in its new form of meeting discharge and bed targets and delivering trained nursing tasks (such as administering drugs) has become a priority, resulting in an increased workload and pace of work and a move away from patient-centred care. Consequently, for the student in 2007, 'the learning is different' and the role of mentor which did not exist for the 1984 student has become of the utmost importance in establishing positive role models and relationships to set the emotional tone and the feeling rules to ensure quality learning and caring. What has also emerged is the importance of the student as the active learner and in particular the recognition among a group of mature students that life experience can play an important part in the 'give and take' or 'the swings and roundabouts' of the mentoring relationship in promoting their emotional wellbeing and learning.

6

Death and dying in hospital: the ultimate emotional labour

Introduction

When I started to update this chapter for the 2010s, as in previous chapters, I began by interrogating the original findings in the context of new research.[1] However, I found that this technique did not work for the topic of death and dying partly because the original chapter had been so tightly argued on the basis of the 1980s data and partly because of my ethnographic experience as a participant observer when I had been so close to the field giving care to patients with student nurses. The follow-up study was also ethnographic in approach and provided the opportunity over a number of weeks to get close to the experience of what it was like to be critically ill in hospital to produce a series of powerful snapshots and stories from students, nurses and teachers about the experience of learning to nurse in the modern NHS. The two studies are presented separately and the findings are then integrated and synthesized in the summary and conclusions.

Defining death and dying in hospitals in the 1980s

The impact of dying in hospital and the feelings surrounding its unsuitability as a place to die struck me the first night I did a night shift early on in the original study. Hannah and Lily were the regular nurses for the shift. I was there as an extra to help out where I could. Although the ward had only 16 beds, at least half the patients were acutely ill. One patient had been admitted following a drug overdose and was being regularly monitored. Another two were receiving treatment for diabetes. Their blood sugar levels, hovering around danger point, were being constantly checked, and their intravenous infusions regulated.

Then there was Mr Brown, who was dying. We were not aware of it at the time. He was old (87), and advanced cancer had left him weak, emaciated and confused. We had been told by the day staff that he was becoming increasingly 'agitated' (a much used convenience label) and noisy. Would we be sure, therefore, to give him his sleeping tablets and pain killers so that he didn't disturb the other patients?

We started off the night shift as usual, doing the routine tasks. There were the medicines to dispense, a complicated ritual of checking and counterchecking for most of the 16 patients. There were also blood pressures to record and temperatures and pulses to take, not to mention the patient or two who called for the commode or for assistance to walk to the bathroom.

Hannah, the staff nurse, asked me to help her with the medicines. When it got to Mr Brown's turn he was in no mood for medicine. He spat most of it out, pushing us away. There was no time for coaxing and cajoling. I remember feeling mildly irritated with the wispy haired, cross old man who was determined not to take the medicine. On reflection, fear rather than 'crossness' was the more likely explanation for Mr Brown's behaviour. We left him to finish the drug round, while Lily, six months into her training, ran between the other patients, helping with toileting and checking the observations of the acutely ill diabetics and the patient who had overdosed.

Lily and I returned to Mr Brown half-an-hour later, but by now he was attempting to get out of bed, nightshirt flapping, and still refusing his medicine. We explained that the medicine was to help him sleep, but he didn't seem to understand. Instead, he muttered incoherently, pushing away the spoon containing the medicine and showing unexpected strength for one so frail looking. I think he thought we might be trying to poison him. It was too late for soothing words, not that either Lily or I felt very calm inside with all the activity and anxiety surrounding the patients with their unstable blood sugars and the man who had taken an overdose beginning to regain consciousness and talk about what he'd done and why.

Finally, Mr Brown, as if worn out with fighting for his life, fell into a fitful sleep. But the anxiety that we felt for the acutely ill patients continued to punctuate the care of Mr Brown all night. We never seemed to have two minutes just to sit with him and calm him and wait with him as he passed from something in between living and dying, a state we were only able to comprehend days later when we returned to the ward to find that he had died. Here was the most profound event of all, and we had not even recognized its imminence in an old man who was strong enough to climb out of bed and push us away. In a ward orientated to acute emergency care and life-threatening situations, Mr Brown's slower, less dramatic, death approached imperceptibly. Our aim that night was to keep him clean and quiet largely for the benefit of the other patients, rather than for his own comfort and safety.

When we found out days later that he was dead we all felt bad that we had let Mr Brown down. The emotional labour we gave felt unsatisfactory and inadequate for someone who we now realized had been dying.

Feelings about death and dying

When during interviews with students during the first study I heard how many of them felt cheated when patients died, I began to understand some of the feelings surrounding Mr Brown's death. The students felt especially cheated if they were off duty when the death occurred. In Mr Brown's case we felt cheated because the last time *we* had seen him he had been in a distressed state. Some days passed before we were on the ward again, and in the meantime he had deteriorated and died. Consequently, we were unable either to improve or to complete the care we had begun.

The students felt cheated especially if the permanent ward staff didn't tell them what had happened to the patient on their return. Not all deaths affected students in this way. But for patients who they had got to know over a period of time and who they felt involved with, being present at their death gave them an opportunity to conclude the care they had begun. For many nurses, closure was attained by performing last offices. I see it as my last duty to them, said one nurse who laid out Mr Owen (aged 50) when treatment for blood cancer finally failed after several weeks in her care.

For those not present at a death, returning to work after a period of absence and not to be told by the trained staff that a patient had died made the students feel doubly cheated. The students believed that the staff's silence represented a failure to recognize the part they had played in the care of the patient and a denial of their right to know that the patient had died. As one student put it 'they just don't want to know'. Another student described the situation in the following way:

> On this ward there's a quick turnover of patients and the thing I particularly noticed when I was on nights that you probably nursed someone for all the time you were on the ward. Then you'd go for your nights off and they could have been discharged. You'd return and you wouldn't know that they had gone and you'd ask the trained staff where they'd gone. They'd just say 'well ... '. Or somebody may have died. Another girl told me she looked after someone for six weeks who died whilst she was on her nights off and she felt cheated that the trained staff hadn't actually told her.

Why did the trained staff seem as if they didn't 'want to know'? One reason was that the students were only allocated to the ward for eight weeks and rarely worked with the same group of staff nurses for any length of time. It was not obvious therefore how the trained staff became aware of how involved students felt about individual patients, nor of their need to know what had happened to those patients while they had been away from the ward. Another reason related to the emotional climate of the ward and whether death and dying were explicit components of the work.[2] On such wards it was usual that students and trained staff had contact with each other both informally, during breaks, and formally, during the ward handover, so that there were opportunities for them to discuss their feelings surrounding patients' deaths.

Some of the best managed deaths were those where the trained staff had known the patients and their families over a period of months and sometimes years. Take David, 45, with a heart condition who had been coming to the same ward for three years. Most of the trained staff had known him for at least a year, when a cure still looked hopeful. Now he was coming into hospital for the last time, to die. I observed that the trained staff used certain strategies to manage David's death. Firstly they decided that only trained staff, the people he knew best, should care for him during his final days and hours. His wife was with him throughout this period, supported by the staff who talked with her and helped her with her husband's care. He was moved to the ward's only single room. One staff nurse who willingly took her turn caring for David said that she hoped she would not be on duty when he died because she felt so sad about his impending death. She was unsure how well she would manage her feelings. On this occasion she was not put to the test. David died several hours after she had gone off duty. The ward sister, on the other hand, who had known David during the three years he had been coming to her ward, asked the staff nurses to ring her at home when his condition deteriorated as she wanted to come into the ward to say goodbye. I found this interesting in that the sister was expressing the need to say goodbye to a patient in the same way as the students. But unlike the students she had both the experience and the control over her work to be able to do that.

Death's unpredictability

Some of the difficulties of managing emotions around death and dying in hospital came from its unpredictability. Students expected from the beginning of training to be called upon to nurse dying patients, resuscitate patients following cardiac arrest and to lay out the dead. Students were ever watchful and sometimes fearful that they might be called upon to cope with death in any of these guises, and saw it as part of their training around which they should acquire specific skills. There were no guarantees, however, that they would meet these situations, as a nurse teacher explained:

> You may well have a student who on her night duty on the ward had a death every night. And you'll find another student who's also worked on the ward and not seen a

dead patient in three years of training. There are students who have been present at at least three or four cardiac arrests. And others who've passed their final exams and never seen one.

And a student said.

When you're a third-year you're expected to have seen most things and done most things. For example: somebody died and sister said to me 'Well I think you can take care of this now'. Neither me nor another third-year had done last offices before. But we wanted to because we thought 'It's about time'. It just happens. You sometimes miss things like that.

As these two accounts demonstrate, the act of death was more readily identified than the process of dying. Death required clearly defined technical skills. If the patient suffered a cardiac arrest, then resuscitation was required. When the patient was pronounced dead then the body had to be laid out.

The point at which patients were recognized as dying, and the skills required to care for them during their transition from life to death were less easy to define, as shown by our experience with Mr Brown. But what the following incident also showed me was that the training needs of students gave them a functional view of death, which in turn could lead to a fragmentation of the patient's technical and emotional care.

Packaging death

John, a 60-year-old man, lay dying of cancer on one of the wards where I had been working. He had been admitted to the ward on previous occasions, but none of the staff he knew were on duty. I had been on the night shift a few hours before he died. He lay with a swollen abdomen and restless. We gave him ice cubes to suck and tried to do what we could to make him physically comfortable, but there was no one around who had actually known him in life, and it seemed a lonely way to go. I heard later how his death had been managed on the following shift. His care was allocated to two students: one in her final year and the other at the beginning of training. Neither student knew John. The management of the death had the feeling of a neat learning package, partly made possible because the students did not feel any emotional attachment to John. The first-year student had not seen anyone die before and was instructed by the third-year student how it should be done. She was instructed to sit with John and hold his hand. As soon as he had died, two third-year students took over and laid him out, because they 'needed the experience'. I found it interesting to observe how the patient's care, by turning it into a sort of 'learning' package for the students, divided the technical from the emotional labour. Even more than that, the emotional labour had been delegated to the most inexperienced nurse of all, i.e. the first-year student.

Following the patient's death, the first-year student had deferred to two senior students who needed to gain experience in laying people out. She had received some acknowledgement for her labour however, when, shortly after John's death, her seniors had asked her how she was feeling. She said she had felt sad but not upset because she did not know the patient well. On overhearing this conversation, I somehow sensed that she said she felt sad because she felt that sadness was an appropriate feeling to feel.[3]

'You knew exactly what to do': a death well managed

Rachel, a student in her first year of training, took part in a patient's death that was managed in an involving and emotionally explicit way. The patient was a Miss Roberts, in her late eighties. She was slowly recovering from bowel surgery, when one morning she woke with excruciating abdominal pain. The doctor was called and X-rays ordered. But there was a long time lapse before she was transferred to the X-ray department, and only mild analgesia was given because of the medical tradition of not wanting to 'mask the pain' before finding its cause. Patients who were Miss Roberts' neighbours told me how Rachel cradled Miss Roberts in her arms, speaking soothingly to her in an effort to comfort her pain.[4]

Miss Roberts was diagnosed as having an inoperable bowel obstruction arising from a postoperative complication. When she returned from having her X-ray she was given stronger pain-killers at last, and she lapsed into semi-consciousness. The staff nurse who was on duty came and sat with Rachel, who remained with Miss Roberts until her sister was called. She died some hours later peacefully, with her sister and Rachel by her side and a vase of her favourite heavily scented flowers on her locker. She was a devout Catholic, and the priest had given her the last rites before she lapsed into unconsciousness. When she had died, the staff nurse asked Rachel whether she felt able to help her lay out Miss Roberts. She readily agreed.

I spoke with Rachel and her friend Jill a few days after Miss Robert's death. Rachel said:

> I got quite attached to Miss Roberts, but she was old and she had to go sometime. It was sad.
>
> PS.   The other patients told me how much you cared for Miss Roberts on her last day.
>
> R.   Well I just realised that she was in total agony.

J.   You knew exactly what to do. You'd nursed her much more than anybody else. You were her nurse.

R.   I don't know.

J.   You did. I didn't know what to do.

R   I suppose I looked after her quite a few times.

This short extract illustrates a number of points. Rachel had formed a relationship with Miss Roberts because she had looked after her a number of times. She therefore knew her quite well, to the extent that Jill saw her as *her* (Miss Roberts') nurse. The staff nurse, recognizing that Miss Roberts was dying, called her relative and clergyman and supported Rachel to complete her care to its natural conclusion. On this occasion, impending death was recognized and prepared for, and holistic rather than packaged care was given.

The technical and emotional labour of death

In some wards, such as the oncology wards, nurses were regularly confronted with death. They became familiar with the technical aspects of laying people out and overcame some of their fears: 'You get to lay out so many people. You know how to do it. It's gruelling, horrible, but I'm not so afraid of death now'.

But as the student also observed: 'One of the problems on a ward like that is you become so blasé. The staff nurses, it's ruining their careers. The involvement with patients becomes too much and they become hard'.

What the student was describing was a process of emotion management by the nurses to distance themselves from patients and the feelings surrounding their deaths. But, as she saw it, becoming blasé and hard as a defence against involvement was ruining their careers. A patient also made a similar observation. She was a 53-year-old care assistant. I was interviewing her to find out her perspectives on nursing, given some of the similarities with her own occupation. She described herself as 'too emotional' to be a nurse. 'It's like when one of my clients dies, it's like losing one of your own'. She paused and reflected: 'Still, some of the nurses must feel the same. But in those cancer wards they must need to change to prevent getting involved'.[5]

The following accounts illustrate why students were concerned with dominating technical skills around the management of death or preventing it, as in the case of cardiac arrest. Night duty was a time when they particularly felt a need for those skills, because it often felt dark and lonely with fewer staff around and patients sleeping.

One student described her first week of night duty on a cancer ward as a junior student. She recounts that she 'hated the whole week of it, but I think I learnt. I think we had two deaths that week and it was quite traumatic, but it built up my confidence'.

Another student, reflecting on her first experience of night duty, said how much she had learnt, particularly when she had witnessed a cardiac arrest. She continued:

> Until then I was afraid of cardiac arrests. It was also the first one for the third-year I was on duty with. The man died. We were both very upset but because I was the first-year I was sent to supper, but nobody supported the third-year. I learnt from that too that third-years still need support.

These accounts suggest that death and cardiac arrest were events that the students feared, but having experienced them gave them the confidence to handle them technically in the future.

What was less obvious was where and how they learnt to manage their emotions around these events. As the last account illustrates, a third-year student was expected to cope, regardless of how inexperienced and upset she felt following a patient's sudden death from cardiac arrest. The student who had shared the experience with her learnt not only technically from the situation about how to manage a cardiac arrest, but also the importance of dealing with the feelings generated from such a stressful event.

Sister Kinder, who was mentioned in Chapter 5 of the first edition, shows us one way in which students can learn to manage their feelings around such events. Following an emergency on her ward, she called students into the day room and discussed the event with them, in order to find out how they were feeling and to reassure them of a job well done.

Although students were grateful for Sister Kinder's recognition of their needs in this informal way, they were doubtful that managing feelings around death and dying could be formally taught. A common view was that 'You can't be taught to react ... if you want to talk about things like death you usually talk about it to your friends when you come off duty'.

Learning about death, like any learning associated with feeling management as expressed in Chapter 3, was seen to be experiential: 'You learn by the way other people do things, like talking to dying patients'.

Then as described in Chapter 4, students were more likely to identify 'terminal care of patients and relatives' as a valuable educational experience on the oncology wards compared with the general medical wards. Yet deaths could occur on any ward at any time. Indeed, many of the accounts of dying presented above were taken from wards other than oncology wards. On these wards, however, the emphasis was much more likely to be on the patient's technical care. Ward tutorials organized by the nurse tutors also tended to concentrate on patients' diseases and treatment. Generally, students preferred it like that. They regarded talking about feelings and attitudes as a waste of time. Occasionally, they mentioned tutorials which addressed the need to do emotional labour and its cost. When they did, as the student illustrates below, these tutorials played an important part in helping students deal with their feelings.

> Yesterday we had a session on the ward with one of the social workers and our tutor. It is very stressful on there because a lot of the patients are young and they are dying of cancer. It was very useful. We could just say what we like and you can realise that it's not just you that feels stressed but probably everyone is feeling the same.

This comment about feeling the same was very important. There was no need for pretence and for being seen to cope when everyone else was feeling the emotion of working in such a stressful environment. The nurses could say how they felt within the confines of the tutorial, allowing them to keep in touch with their feelings when they returned to the public arena.

Death and bereavement

I am now going to tell two stories about two different patients on two different wards. The stories have some striking similarities. They are stories about elderly patients, both of whom were bereaved of close relatives and one of whom faced his own death. The key people who cared for them were student nurses in their first few months of training. The student nurses were very much in touch with what the patients were going through, but had no arena in which to work on those feelings and emotions.

The first story concerns Mr Lawrence, a man in his eighties. Mr Lawrence was admitted from his local hospital for a palliative procedure to relieve the large tumour in his common bile duct. The tumour was causing a damming up of bile, and by the time he was admitted to the ward his skin had turned a profound yellow. Mr Lawrence looked heavy and uncomfortable. His skin itched from the bile pigments, and he complained of nausea and not being able to eat. He looked very miserable and withdrawn. Because he hadn't officially been told of his diagnosis, it was presumed that he didn't know that he had cancer. Judging from his facial expressions and behaviour, I doubted somehow that he didn't know. Soon after admission Mr Lawrence's son died suddenly of a heart attack. Mr Lawrence drew into himself even further, lying silently on his bed with the curtains drawn around him. We were told in the ward report by the trained staff that he did not wish to attend his son's funeral. Again I wondered how much of this was based on assumptions and superficial discussions.

On this ward, it was very much the trained staff who controlled communication and exchange of information. A comment in my field notes during this period reads: 'A very silent exchange: nurses with heads down scribbling; only trained staff giving information. Few comments made by students. For feedback, trained staff asked to be notified of any changes in patients' conditions'.

Not surprisingly, it was difficult to work out from these ward handover reports just how much real assessment of Mr Lawrence's emotional state had taken place.

The trained staff acknowledged in the handover reports that Mr Lawrence was depressed following his son's death. The nurses were instructed to 'chat' to him. There was no discussion or guidance about how to do this and what to say.

When Jane, one of the staff nurses, told me how difficult it was to talk to Mr Lawrence, I began to understand why the students were not being given any better guidance than to 'chat' to him. She explained that whenever she attempted to talk to him he started crying. 'I just avoid him now', she said. Jane was not an unkind person; she just found difficulties talking to people about their feelings. She liked to get on with what she saw as the 'real' work of the ward: the bedbaths, the dressings and the medications. It was interesting that when I left the ward at the end of fieldwork, she thanked me for being an extra pair of hands.

On talking to Lorraine, a first-year student nurse, about Mr Lawrence she told me just how helpless she had felt to support him. After about 12 days in the hospital the doctors decided that as Mr Lawrence did not seem to be making any progress, he'd better be transferred back to his local hospital. This was often the pattern with patients who had come from other hospitals for specific treatments. If it looked as if they might die, the doctors made hurried arrangements to get them off the ward. It was as if they did not want to have a patient who had not responded to their treatment dying on them. It was almost as if Mr Lawrence decided that he couldn't face another move. The night following the doctors' decision to transfer him to his home hospital, Mr Lawrence began to vomit blood, and within hours he was dead. That night, Lorraine was on the night shift. This is what she said about him:

> From the moment I nursed him, he just wanted to give up life altogether; he was very apathetic, I'd say. There was nothing you could do. I used to go and sit and talk to him if I had time, but he was just not willing to talk, he wasn't one of those patients who bottled everything up and then came out with it. He just gave one word answers all the time and you felt you weren't getting anywhere and you felt: well, he was eighty or whatever and it's his choice really. I've always heard that people could give up and just turn their backs or whatever, but that's a real classic case.

Lorraine described her efforts to help Mr Lawrence, but to no avail because she felt: 'He was just rejecting me totally, and you felt as if you were imposing on his privacy. He kept the curtains half drawn as well. I always felt this is not my position to come here'.

I knew how she felt. I had had the same feelings when trying to talk to Mr Lawrence myself, as had Jane, the staff nurse who had started avoiding him when every time she talked to him he began to cry. Lorraine had recognized the need to do emotional labour for Mr Lawrence, but had lacked guidance and support on how to manage her feelings and the feelings that he generated.

Lorraine and Jane clearly felt dissatisfied with the way in which they had managed Mr Lawrence's emotional care. Jane withdrew her emotional labour by avoiding him. Lorraine felt rejected, and believed the patient had given up the will to live, so excusing her from 'imposing on his privacy'.

The final story concerns Jill, a student on her first ward. Her work as an au pair with a family where the mother of young children was dying of cancer had prepared her for dealing with issues around death and dying. She was surprised, therefore, on her first placement, a cardiology ward, to find that the ward staff didn't expect her to be interested in people. She said:

> I'm much more interested in the social side of things, making patients happy like Bridget ... there should be someone who can sort things out for her, sort out what's going round in her head.

Bridget was an elderly patient who had been admitted to the ward when her husband had died suddenly from a stroke. She was suffering from Parkinson's disease and was sometimes forgetful. She had been pronounced 'unable to cope alone at home', since her husband had been the main care giver. I met her on the morning after her admission. She was small and slim with shoulder-length hair, a wide friendly mouth and large spectacles. She walked with the shuffling gait typical of Parkinson's disease. Bridget was warm and open and said what she felt. Even though she was 67 years old she had a childlike manner, which probably came from years of being cared for by her husband. They had no children. When she spoke of him, Bridget's eyes filled with tears, saying how good he had been to her and what she was going to do without him. She referred to him as 'daddy'. Many of the students presumed that Bridget was confusing her husband with her father and took this as a sign that she was demented. This wasn't so. Bridget, like many elderly working class couples, especially those without children, referred to their spouse as 'mum' or 'dad'. Bridget was shocked and disorientated by her husband's death, but she wasn't demented.

I noticed that student Jill talked a lot with Bridget. They sat closely together at the end of Bridget's bed talking at some length. Jill was quietly attentive with head inclined and eyes closely focused on Bridget.

There was some confusion about whether Bridget should go to her husband's funeral or not. The general line on the ward was that she did not want to go, but Jill had other opinions, based on her many discussions with Bridget. During the ward report, Jill told me that she had tried to make Bridget's wishes known to the trained staff. They responded by looking surprised at her intervention and turning their attention to the nurse who was in charge of the shift as if seeking more reliable information. In the end Bridget did get to her husband's funeral, but Jill was not satisfied at the way it had been managed. She described the circumstances to me:

> I was really quite upset about Bridget's husband's funeral. I found that very frustrating, whisked off at the last minute. I actually said to one of the staff nurses 'She does want to go you know' and she said 'we've asked her and she doesn't'. But I said 'she just told me and she wants to go'. And I thought well I have no say in it. And suddenly there was a great drama and laughs and giggles and she was got off at the last minute in a taxi. It was a mess but I couldn't do anything about it.

As in the case of Mr Lawrence, the enormity of bereavement had not been discussed among the ward staff. The person who had invested the most emotional labour in helping her to sort out her feelings about going to the funeral was Jill, a first-year student. Jill felt she had been regarded as too junior to be taken seriously by the trained staff and helpless to intervene. Neither had she been allowed to accompany Bridget to the funeral. The staff had finally taken on board that Bridget wanted to go to the funeral, but Jill felt they had handled it badly. They turned their last-minute decision into a 'drama' with laughs and giggles, possibly to hide their own embarrassment as well as to distract attention from the sadness of the occasion.

Bridget's situation is reminiscent of Mr Lawrence's. It was reported that he did not want to go to his son's funeral. Similarly, Bridget was said not to want to go to her husband's funeral. Jill invested emotional labour and elicited an opposite response to the official one. But Bridget welcomed the opportunity to talk about her feelings. Lorraine described the difficulty of caring for Mr Lawrence. Unlike Bridget he was withdrawn and remote. He made Lorraine feel that she was invading on his privacy and was reluctant to talk.

Both these stories illustrate the sensitivity of the first-year students to their own and their patients' feelings. But the feeling rules of the wards were bounded by a rigid nursing hierarchy, which operated in two ways. Firstly, it kept the feelings associated with death and dying in place by failing to acknowledge them in the public arena of the ward handovers. Secondly, the trained staff made Lorraine and Jill feel, because of their junior status, that their opinions and views about patients would not be taken seriously.

Both students had important insights on the emotional state of the two patients. In Lorraine's view, Mr Lawrence decided to die. But if her insights had been shared, the way in which he died might have been managed in a more emotionally sustaining way for both nurses and patient. Jill too felt that there was nothing she could have done to avoid the 'mess' surrounding Bridget's husband's funeral. I wondered how long Lorraine and Jill would retain their emotional sensitivity in a hierarchy that neither acknowledged nor sustained it.

The role of the hierarchy in managing death

The hierarchy on many wards kept students and trained staff very separate from each other. They inhabited two different worlds and developed separate sets of social relations with the patients. The trained staff were more likely to get to know and invest in the deaths of the patients that had been coming to their ward over time. The students became involved with patients they had nursed during their eight-week placement. Common to both groups was that nurses did not feel the same way about the death and dying of all their patients but only those with whom they had formed a relationship, usually over time.

The hierarchy also served to separate technical from emotional labour by dictating that, at certain stages of training, students should be able to perform specific technical tasks around death and dying, such as cardiopulmonary resuscitation and last offices.

There was also an expectation that the more senior a student was the more likely she would be expected to cope with upsetting situations. It seemed that because students' feelings were rarely acknowledged in the open arena of the ward that they were likely to develop distancing strategies which kept them from personal involvement. They recognized that, as they progressed through their careers, they might become hard. But they also recognized that if they hardened and distanced too much they would be unable to nurse with feeling.

On the other hand, they were unwilling to believe that they could learn to 'react'. They preferred to see learning about feelings and emotions associated with death and dying as experiential: going through the experiences themselves and observing what other people did. Their reluctance to recognize the skill of learning and how to manage complex feelings was bound up with the way in which death and dying were defined in hospitals according to the patient's diagnosis and the feeling rules of the ward determined by the medical speciality, the hierarchy and the ward sister's work preferences and priorities.

Facing death and dying in the 2000s

So what is the situation as we enter the second decade of the twenty-first century? Would Mr. Brown, whom I describe at the beginning of this chapter, fare any better now? Our fieldwork observations in 2007 revealed detailed data about advanced old age and the dilemmas faced by elderly patients and their families as they were admitted to acute hospitals with fractures or infections over and above the chronic conditions such as dementia, Congestive Cardiac Failure (CCF) or Chronic Obstructive Pulmonary Disease (COPD) that they were already suffering from. During fieldwork on an orthopaedic ward for example, I heard about the patient who desperately wanted to go home but was deemed unsafe to do so by the ward staff, because only limited care could be provided by social services. We also listened during interviews and focus groups to what the students and their teachers had to say about the care of older and dying people on the wards and in the community in their own or residential homes and hospices.

I concluded from these data to broaden the scope of the original chapter 6 to address not only the final phase of dying but the long journey that often precedes it. For older people in particular, this journey was often characterized by multiple hospital admissions, periods of rehabilitation, gradual loss of independence, a mix of residential care homes, hospices, community health and social care and the heartbreaking realization on the part of the patient (and also family and friends, staff and students) that they would not recover. Holman (2008) worked with staff caring for dependent older people in a continuing care environment where she found that the theme of loss emerged as central to the work. The phrase 'living bereavement' was devised, which covered the complex feelings associated with witnessing the cumulative loss of older people as they slowly declined from one acute crisis to the next against a background of chronic illness.[6]

Student responses to the ward learning environment questionnaire described the emotional demands of nursing and in some instances gave examples of the stress and anxiety associated with nursing sick and dying patients. They wrote of their stress and anxiety when staffing levels were so low that they felt unable to provide patients with the quality or the quantity of the care they required. The students also wrote of their need to be adequately supported by the qualified staff to manage the ultimate emotional labour of caring for patients who were dying but also the aftermath of their death.

Since the publication of the first book, death and dying have become popular media topics with articles, news coverage and television programmes abounding. The death of celebrities, particularly young ones like Princess Diana 'The People's Princess' in 1997, resulted in enormous manifestations of public grief and a decade later 'Reality TV' star Jade Goody, who was suffering from cervical cancer, allowed her final days and hours to be publicly broadcast. Described as a 'tragic heroine of our time', Goody has become the 'perfect subject' for a high profile play (Brooks 2011).

The increase in the number of journalists who are either going through the experience of caring for ageing and ailing parents and/or growing older themselves may explain why end-of-life issues as a media topic has increased in popularity. Joan Bakewell, a prominent journalist, who at the age of 75 was appointed as an 'independent and informed advocate' and 'Voice of Older People' is able to raise issues and represent the interests of her many peers who live active and independent lives into extreme old age.

But there are still people like Mr. Brown who frequently appear in the acute wards during their final days. The chances that they will receive appropriate care during this time have been improved by the introduction in 2007 of the Liverpool Care

Pathway for the Dying Patient (LCP) in recognition of the increased need for palliative care in acute care settings for people with cancer and other conditions. The purpose of the pathway is 'to provide an evidence based framework for the delivery of appropriate care for dying patients and their relatives in a variety of settings'.[7]

As if to bear this out a moving account described as 'care among the chaos' in the *Guardian* newspaper of 23 October 2007 portrayed the last days of a much cherished mother who died in her own home surrounded by her family and supported by regular visits from carers, district nurses and their teams.

But death is still much more likely to take place in hospital rather than home, hospice or residential home[8] because even cancer, like other long-term conditions can be unpredictable, often making the final trajectory, the death watch and the need for the ultimate emotional labour difficult to define and recognize.

Death and dying have always been popular topics for ethnographers, and since the 1980s an increasing number of researchers have built on the classic works of Fox (1959), Glaser and Strauss (1965), Quint (1967) and Sudnow (1967). Nicky James (1986) explicitly connected care, emotions and work in nursing the dying, closely followed by David Field (1989), Jo Hockey (1990) and Julia Lawton (2000). Lawton studied patients' experiences of palliative care and the dying process in a hospice. Her analysis revealed the 'messiness' of dying, categorized at its extreme as 'dirty dying'. The power of this category as a descriptor was reminiscent of the following account of working with a student to care for an extremely debilitated elderly woman suffering the dual indignities of a large sacral ulcer and frequent incontinence. My co-researcher Helen graphically describes nursing the patient in the hot, cramped conditions of a busy medical ward in a large district hospital. Helen wrote:

> 07.45, and it's very busy, linen bags, sheets etc all down the corridor; doctors, nurses darting in and out of bays. Sister greeted me with open arms! First year student was working with sister but very busy ward and patients in one bay needed full washes/bed baths. We set to ... second patient was confused, had kept the bay awake by shouting, smelt of faeces and needed a full bed bath. Student went to gather things we'd need and we started. The woman had a big sacral sore, necrotic and 'dirty' with faeces. The bed bath took about 45 minutes; it was hot, smelly, and difficult to move the woman and the student was unsure of herself. However the woman kept saying 'thank you' and looked better afterwards; she then went on to be incontinent of faeces ten minutes later.

Once having made the patient comfortable again, Helen and the student went for a coffee break and asked her how she was feeling. The student replied:

> Oh you just get on with it. I've never seen anything like that before but I have now and it's fine. I just think if you can help someone, like we were, she kept saying we were, then that's okay.

The student then went on to describe a situation that she had found difficult to deal with emotionally. She said:

> Before Christmas there was a man with very painful legs, they were falling apart and he was in pain. I couldn't do anything and I found that difficult, to see someone come in and then in a week, like that go downhill and die. We couldn't help. That's what I found difficult when I'm not in control. The other stuff is okay because we can do something about it.

Helen asked the student whether she had talked to anybody about how she had felt. The student replied:

> Well all the staff were really upset too. The other student in my cohort and I were holding his hands and trying to reassure him and it was upsetting – there was nothing we could do.

Helen also asked her if she talked to her friends about her experience but the student replied:

> No I don't see them during placement and I live at home. We have reflection at college and sometime talk about what we've done. But I didn't with that one, no.

This experience made a big impression on Helen because of the extremes of emotions that the staff had to cope with. Yet these emotions would have gone largely unexpressed partly because there did not appear to be any structured opportunities for reflection and partly because the ward (and therefore the staff) was very busy. When it came to the students there was no longer any sense of them sitting together talking through the shift.

Death and dying – still the ultimate emotional labour

In 2007 the findings quickly revealed that death and its impact on the caring and learning experience is no less significant than it was in the 1980s, even though there is now more public recognition of end-of-life processes. As mentioned above, current students' responses to the ward learning environment questionnaires revealed not only the emotional demands and 'consequences' of nursing sick and dying patients as a source of stress but also the support necessary to assist them to manage the ultimate emotional labour. As one student commented 'lack of support from members of staff when there was a death on the ward' led her to question just as her 1980s predecessor had before her[9] that 'Nobody asked if I was ok, or if I had any questions, or if I needed to talk to anyone about what had happened'.

Further findings suggest that one reason why this perceived lack of support persists may be because the 'busyness' of the current NHS ward environment puts pressure on ward managers and staff to meet targets and manage a fast patient throughput, creating stress for all nurses both trained assistants and students alike. Taylor (2006) argues that the emotional toil of caring for people in sickness and as they die is rarely referred to in policy, yet the emotional effect of working with sick patients and their relatives captured by Holman (2008) as 'living bereavement' was clearly evident in our fieldwork. Participant observation in particular showed how present and yet how uncontained emotions were for student nurses. Helen recorded the following incident in her field notes:

> It was a gynae-oncology ward and on that shift there were two patients dying aged between 35–40 years old and another patient who had come back to the ward in shock and was being resuscitated; the curtains were drawn around her and one of the Sisters kept going in and out. The shift started at 07.45 when the sister, staff nurses and the health care assistants (HCAs) emerged from handover followed by two very hesitant students who hung around looking uncertain. Eventually after the staff nurses started the drug rounds on both sides of the ward, the students started giving out breakfasts. I approached the Sister and she asked me to go and find the students which I did. We then made beds, did a dressing and observations. I later went for coffee with one second year and one third year student. As we sipped our coffee the second year student asked me if I'd always enjoyed nursing and I said that I had. I then asked her how she was finding it. She said:

> It's been difficult, shocking coming into nursing from school; the amount of work you have to do....

> The third year student then joined in and said that she found:

> The stress and psychological [effect] builds up and feels heavy on your shoulders until you explode which is what I did the day before with the practice educator.

The problem as she explained it to Helen seemed to be that as a senior third year student she did not feel that she had had sufficient nursing experience to register as a qualified nurse in the near future, and she had directed her stress at the practice educator. The student in this instance had been unable to contain her emotions, nor undertake emotional labour to suppress them so that she 'exploded' at her teacher. Now she was directing her anxiety and frustration at Helen with the assertion that:

> I know we have to do washes, beds, breakfasts, observations – but when the trained staff do drugs they should call me to look and learn. But they don't! I qualify in a month and I won't be able to do anything as a nurse.

This third year student's reaction was similar to how third-year students reacted in the first study, who also said they felt inadequately prepared to practise as qualified nurses because of a lack of exposure to what they perceived to be key technical skills essential for the job.

Helen further speculated that because of the stress on the ward arising from seriously ill and dying patients the staff nurses were undertaking the drug rounds on their own as a means of containing their own anxiety and distress while leaving the students to get on with the patients' personal care which were judged to be within their capabilities and therefore did not require them to be directly supervised. The consequence for the students was that it put them in direct contact with physically and emotionally distressed patients, so although they had not been allocated to care for the critically ill and dying women on the ward, this situation undoubtedly created an emotionally charged atmosphere which required the ultimate emotional labour. In the acute hospital ward, targets to speed up patient throughput leaves little space for emotional engagement. Consequently, staff nurses undertake the technical tasks to get the work done which may act as a mechanism to contain their feelings and reduce their direct engagement with both students and patients. Put another way, the feelings are passed down to the students to directly engage in the ultimate emotional labour of end-of-life care.

Students' stories in the 2000s

Stories captured during interviews with student nurses revealed that similar end-of-life issues in relation to the ultimate emotional labour evident in the first study persist. Such issues include knowing what to do when a patient is critically ill or dying, being supported to know what to do for patients at the end of life, the expectation that students should have 'seen most things and done most things' by their third year of training, the acute hospital ward as an unsuitable place to die; packaging death and the interface between caring and nursing. I now present a number of student stories which capture some of these issues.

'No one to help when your first patient dies'

Miriam was a third year student nearing the end of her three-year diploma programme. She had had a busy morning shift and came directly from the acute ward to be interviewed in the education centre about a ten-minute walk from the clinical areas. She immediately started talking about dealing with emergencies particularly now that she was in her final module before qualifying. She described how during a recent shift, a patient she was caring for had suddenly collapsed. Her allocated mentor was nowhere to be found. Miriam said that as she had deliberately organized her shifts to coincide with her mentor's roster, she had felt very let down when she discovered she was not on the ward but was attending a training course. She then described going from one trained member of staff to another asking for help only to be told they were all too busy. Miriam had found this situation particularly upsetting because she looked to her mentor to provide someone 'you can go to if you have problems or if you need support, like when your first patient dies, or collapses'. Miriam added she found it hard to switch off once 'off duty' because she continued to feel responsible for her patients. Miriam thought this was partly because she did not always have the chance to debrief with her mentor and 'hand over' her responsibilities before going off the shift. She found this surprising compared with her previous career experience in the customer services department of a large bank, where the mentoring role had been well recognized.

'Talking and cups of tea'

Janet, a second year student, described her work in a hospice as a pre-nursing student, as 'talking and cups of tea'. But now as a student nurse, although she was able to see that these activities were important, she also recognized that 'you need the personal care, like helping people to wash; washing is quite personal'. In this case, Janet was seeing 'personal care' as skilled work which complemented the 'making of cups of tea'. Put another way, in the British culture the cup of tea is very important for creating the opportunity to talk and off load as the Marie Curie advert (which I describe in Chapter 1) drew attention to in the 1990s.

Clearly, Janet's earlier experiences still featured in her view of nursing. When for example I asked her whether she was beginning to identify particular types of nursing she preferred, she replied 'palliative care' because she liked the continuity of seeing familiar faces of both patients and their relatives. Janet added that she had also enjoyed her community placements because 'you could get to know the patient better, and on their terms as you were visiting them in their own homes'. For Janet, relationships were clearly an important aspect of nursing.

She then described a recent hospital experience of caring for a frightened 'elderly lady' with dementia. Janet had subsequently been told by a relative that 'the way you held her hand; how you helped with her feeding made all the difference'. Janet also tried to understand why the old lady scratched and grabbed at the nurses, guessing it was her response to fear and disorientation like Mr. Brown's reactions all those years ago.

I later observed Janet and her mentor working together on a busy orthopaedic ward preparing elderly patients for theatre. Janet's mentor was a good role model. While preparing for surgery a frail elderly lady with dementia and a hip fracture, the mentor calmed the patient by a combination of administering oxygen and soothing words. Moving on to the next patient Janet spotted that she was hard of hearing. Even though the patient was only minutes from being transferred to the theatres, and had been stripped of all aids, Janet reinserted the patient's hearing aid until the moment just prior to anaesthesia as a way of improving communication and reducing anxiety. I speculated that Janet was able to take this action because of the caring, calming, measured approach to patients demonstrated by her mentor and probably because of her previous experience of caring for older, distressed people.

'I'd never done care work before'

Rose was a second year student nurse who described herself as 'very keen' and 'quite passionate' about the care of older people. She identified 'care in the community' as 'the big one' for promoting older people's 'independence' as well as caring for the dying when the time came whether at home, hospital or residential home. Prior to commencing her nursing programme, Rose had worked in a residential home. This experience had been very important to her because she had 'never done care work before'. She said the experience had given her 'confidence' to meet people, make relationships and get to know them. She believed that gaining experience of care work in the calmer context of a residential home had assisted her to make relationships and get to know people in the 'busy' environment of the NHS.

Rose also talked about the difference of caring for people in the NHS compared with the residential home and in particular what she had experienced as the unsatisfactory nature of 'end-of-life' care on the wards, where older people were often regarded as 'bed blockers'. Rose recalled many cases of older patients who needed to be transferred to a nursing home or even their own home when they most needed it as a more suitable place to die than an acute hospital ward. But if they were to die in hospital then Rose was of the opinion that they should be nursed in a side ward where they could be given the attention they needed. Rose added: 'you can't be too specific when they come in to hospital: it's just got to be patient-centred care'. This view was interesting in that she was promoting patient centredness off her own bat which contrasted with the student in the first study who raised the question as to whether hospitals could be geared to each person or not (see Chapter 5).[10]

Given the even greater emphasis on a 'technical-economic' rationality (Davies 1990) underpinning the organization of hospital care in the 2000s and indicated by targets, the student retained a sense of her own role in patient care and how as a nurse she could make a difference. She told me about the feedback given to her by an elderly patient on the point of discharge, who said she'd watched her at work and how she gave: 'a smile, a hug…. I've watched you… you'll make a good nurse'.

Emerging from these accounts is the sense that care is seen as distinct from nursing and that the nursing home, hospice or the patient's own home provides a more appropriate environment to care for the dying than the 'busyness' of the NHS. Care involves emotional labour to make relationships and get to know people, which in turn give students confidence to operate within the target-driven environment of the NHS.

New ways of packaging death

During the first study I recall a stricken relative telling me that she had arrived too late to be with her father when he died. But she had felt some comfort to be told that 'there was someone with him when he died'. Allocating a nurse to sit with a dying patient was very much in keeping with the tradition predominant in the 1980s that no patient was left to die alone. Often the most junior nurse was asked to perform this last duty and did it well. As I observed during the first study, when students were not emotionally attached to patients they might parcel up the different aspects of the dying process in order to care for them and gain essential experience.

In the subsequent study, allocating students to sit with dying patients no longer appeared to be common practice in the acute settings where we undertook our fieldwork. When asking why this may be, it was attributed to 'speed up' and high throughput of patients as well as the students' supernumerary status, which encouraged them to focus on achieving their learning objectives during their placements – hence this could explain the feeling described by the student working with Helen that she was 'wasting' time if she had not had the opportunity to undertake what she and her colleagues saw as 'nursing' rather than caring tasks during the shift.

Furthermore, many nurse managers on the acute wards were so focused on patient discharge that death and dying did not automatically feature as part of their discourse. In Chapter 5, one manager described how her role had changed following the introduction of targets to maintain high bed occupancy and throughput in the NHS, requiring her to become more outward looking and externally focused than in the first 20 years of her career. Indeed she would have been a contemporary of the ward sisters in the first study. She said:

> I've been a ward sister in different guises since the early 80s and initially it was ward focused and it was patient focused and training staff and student focused and that's where your work lay but now the priorities have changed...

So the hypothesis to emerge from these findings is that in the new NHS, there is no place in the 'speed up' target-driven culture to cope with the horror and messiness of extreme illness so that the chronically ill patient may slip at any time across the border from living to dying. Also the introduction of the Liverpool Care Pathway (LCP) may have become a modern way of packaging death to manage its unpredictability and provide a distancing device to defend against the practitioner's anxiety. That the LCP may have unintended consequences was brought to my attention by Helen who described a discussion with her personal student group. She was shocked to hear how they described patients 'being put on LCP's to die' so that rather than being the 'dying patient' they became the 'LCP'. Helen speculated that the LCP was being used as a mechanism to help students keep death at a distance and give them a sense of control rather than the intuitive way Rachel, a young student in my first study, appeared to care for Miss Roberts. The need to feel in control is a theme already highlighted by the student who described to Helen the experience of caring for the man with the 'very painful legs' for whom she felt she 'couldn't do anything'.

Caring not nursing

During fieldwork, I observed an elderly woman, who I will call Edna, who was suffering from pneumonia and advanced congestive cardiac failure, and she was clearly dying. There was no one with her as she lay drifting in and out of the twilight world between life and death. Sometimes she was restless, other times seemingly asleep but then suddenly woke with a start, calling out for her sister, her husband, her mother. She was in a six-bedded bay, and there was no attempt to screen her bed from the other women contrary to Rose's view that dying patients should have a side room and not be nursed in the public gaze of the general ward. However for Edna being in the ward surrounded by kind, wise women in their late middle age turned out to be a better alternative to the seclusion of a side ward. The women recognized her anguish and sat with her, providing a comforting presence. The nurses were noticeable by their absence. The women were not impressed. The health care assistants did what they could but they worked to routines. Edna clearly needed their attention first as they began the morning washes on what was to be her last day on this earth. But she was number three in the row, and she had to wait her turn. Eventually she had her wash and was turned and refreshed with a clean gown and her hair brushed but there was no sense that she was given the care of the dying. She was just another patient in a bed who needed her morning wash when her turn came. On the other hand the women knew and they never left her, taking it in turns to sit and hold her hand or speak comforting words until her family came and took over the death watch of their own accord. That Edna was dying had never been formally acknowledged by the nursing and health care staff. But at least the other patients had sensed her situation, and she was with her family when she died.

One hypothesis to emerge from these accounts is to suggest that on account of speed up and routinization of care, tasks have been carved up between health care assistants, who do the personal care, and nurses, who undertake technical tasks. When student nurses were apprentices they would undertake the full spectrum of care including the personal tasks and the care of the dying. So in the case of Rachel, the traditional task of the junior student nurse apprentice was to give personal care to patients and through that experience learn 'what to do' at the extremes of care. For the modern day student nurse, caught between personal care and technical tasks on the one hand and health care assistant and qualified nurse roles on the other, the care of the dying may get lost in the 'busyness' of routines and targets of the modern NHS. Furthermore the registered nurses feel under great pressure to complete these routines and targets. The LCP offers both a promise and a challenge to care of the dying in 'mainstream settings' and to recognize and support the ultimate emotional labour required.

Summary

When I started to update this chapter for the 2010s I found that the technique of interrogating the original findings in the same manner as in previous chapters did not work for the topic of death and dying. This was partly because the original chapter had been so tightly argued on the basis of the 1980s data and the ethnographic experience of participant observation close to the field. The ethnographic field work for the subsequent study, although conducted over weeks rather than months, did however give the opportunity to generate a series of powerful stories which illustrated the marked division that had emerged between nursing and caring articulated in the 1980s as the interface between technical, physical and affective care and ascribed to year of student nurse training rather than grade of staff.

So the impact that this division had on the students' experience of undertaking the ultimate emotional labour to manage death and dying during student nurse training in the 2000s was that they are now more on the side lines looking in, unlike Rachel 'who had really known what to do' to care for Miss Roberts in her death agony.

A number of changes in relation to common perceptions of death and dying were observed to have entered the public gaze in terms of reality TV and the prominence given to older celebrities as ambassadors of their peers. Another change has been the success of treatments in the management of long-term conditions so that many of the illnesses that were regarded as acute and imminently terminal such as cancers, HIV/AIDS, cardiovascular and pulmonary conditions can now be managed in many cases into extreme old age.

The dying trajectory is therefore less easy to predict but when death comes it may still be unpredictable, unexpected and difficult to manage in an acute hospital setting. New approaches to death and dying such as the LCP, while helping to raise the visibility of death and the need to manage dying sensitively and carefully may also have been used in some cases as a potential device to distance emotional involvement with patients and their families. The potential of the hospice and care home as places where students may be supported to understand their role in assisting people to come to terms with long-term disability and the realization that although death is not imminent they will never recover from their long-term condition, also needs to be recognized in terms of 'living bereavement' (Holman 2008).

In comparison the 'busyness' of the current NHS environment puts pressure on ward managers and staff to meet targets and manage a fast patient throughput in the acute wards, which may mean they are geared to discharge rather than death and dying as visible components and outcomes of the workload. Students are caught in the gap as mentors struggle to care for patients at the same time as caring for students. The feeling rules of the ward therefore are about getting patients through to discharge at the potential expense of the students' learning and emotional needs. In Chapter 7 I examine how this dilemma may be resolved as the students negotiate their way through a modern caring trajectory and the acquisition of caring styles and capacity over their three-year programme.

The caring trajectory: caring styles and capacity over time

My research in the 1980s showed that the 'ideal' nurse or ward sister had a 'caring side'. She put people first and organized her work in an emotionally explicit way to make others feel safe and cared for. Not all nurses chose to organize their work in this way, but preferred to focus on tasks and hierarchy which made others feel anxious and defensive. What happened to students' caring styles and capacity to care during their three-year training, and what were the factors that shaped their emotional careers?

The three-year nurse education programme featured in the second study was a different emotional experience for the students from the outset. Their expectations as supernumerary students were different in that they no longer considered themselves to be part of the official workforce. As we saw in previous chapters, both staff and students interpreted supernumerary status in a variety of ways. Inevitably with the demands of rapid patient turnover and throughput, direct patient care took precedence over student learning. Students described the consequences:

> I was told on my first day on the ward that I would be used in the numbers as the work load is heavy and there is not enough staff

Or:

> The staff were so busy they did not have time for the students, so we were just used as an extra number and I did not feel I learnt as much as I could have

Another student even went so far as to describe her ward experience as 'more about beds than patients', which was a stark example of the target-driven culture which put staff under pressure to get patients in and out of hospital as quickly as possible so that they ended up managing beds rather than people.

Students had a range of competing commitments as they navigated their three-year trajectory of learning objectives, outcomes and 'paperwork' that had to be checked at the beginning, midpoint and end of their placements when their mentors had to officially sign them off as competent. One student described her learning as a bit of 'a gamble', giving the sense that the content of the placements could be unpredictable and reliant on the type of patients admitted to the ward at any one time but constrained by the formal academic criteria set out in the curriculum. She said:

> A placement on an acute medical ward was great to learn about all sorts of medical procedures although sometimes hard to meet all the criteria required for essays and portfolios. It is a bit of a gamble and dependent on which treatments patients require at the time of placements as to whether you are able to use them as evidence to meet the learning criteria. If you don't come across a patient with the issues you need to address for the work needed for essays and portfolios it can be a bit of a problem.

Another student felt that sometimes module learning outcomes were unable to be achieved in some placements as:

> ...They do not have the facilities or staff to enable this. I feel that placements should be thought of in relation to modules and as to whether they are suitable for an individual at a particular stage of training, such as giving a first year nurse (with no previous training) a first placement in A&E.

This comment is also in line with the views of students in the first study about the types of placement they deemed were more suitable than others at different stages of their training. For example busy acute wards and departments (such as A&E) were not seen as suitable at the beginning of their programme. One student who had just completed a placement on a busy surgical ward advised her lecturers not to send 'first year students on such a busy ward as most of them will drop out by the end of the placement'.

For another student on a busy surgical ward even at the beginning of her programme, there was an expectation that 'delivering basic care' would not fulfil her learning outcomes, whereas another first year student did not hold this view. On the contrary all experiences were learning for her:

> As a first year student I found that most experiences involved a degree of useful learning. Perhaps I was lucky with the ward I was on.

This comment suggested, as I found in the first study, that the creation of the learning environment depended not only on the learning material available on the ward ('most experiences involved a degree of useful learning') but also on the way in which the trained staff made the learning accessible ('perhaps I was lucky with the ward I was on').

One final year student was concerned to:

Seek out the critical situations as these are vital learning opportunities. On my most recent placement I was provided with situations where I was able to observe and practise nursing critical patients.

She also maintained that:

Nursing patients who require a basic level of nursing care is not really beneficial to a final year student who already has the basics of nursing under his or her belt. This should be understood and taken into consideration by the mentors on the ward so as to make the learning environment as beneficial to the student as possible so as to graduate with a sound level of understanding and continue to seek out further learning opportunities as a staff nurse.

Another third year student close to the end of her programme was concerned that:

I have had limited ward experience. I feel that a five week placement in a nursing home at this stage in my training is inappropriate as learning opportunities are limited.

Nursing home experience was seen as more appropriate for first-year placements when, as described in Chapter 4, students learnt the confidence to operate in busy NHS settings. Personal care generally was no longer valued as part of a qualified nurse's repertoire.

The students also described the 'amount of academic work' that they were required to undertake as competing with the demands of their placements, which in effect they regarded as holding down a 'fulltime job'. Many students also took part-time employment to supplement their bursaries and particularly those who were mature students, saw this as essential to meet their family commitments.

One student described how hard it was being the 'new student' evoked by the emotional demands of frequently changing wards and moving to new placements. She clearly recognized the emotional labour involved in needing to make an effort to 'show eagerness to learn, work and fit in with ALL the ward staff' on the one hand but who in return she found to be 'generally kind and considerate' of her needs.

The student nurse trajectory in the 1980s

The student experience in the first study was based on an apprenticeship style of training in which they spent the majority of their time moving through the wards, departments and community settings associated with one school of nursing. There was also a clear demarcation between the years as they progressed from their first year of training to the specialities in their second year and on to the demands and challenges of being a third year student. Each year was characterized by an expectation embedded in the folklore of student nurse training from first-year students who were 'so good to have around' to the third year 'blues time' when students were at risk of becoming depressed, disillusioned and cynical. These characterizations, which seemed particular to the first study, and the apprenticeship style of training are revisited below.

First-year students: 'so good to have around'

Students believed that they changed during their training. They came into nursing fresh and enthusiastic, but by the end of three years they had become cynical and disillusioned. They remembered with nostalgia their first year and looked to the current juniors who were 'so good to have around'.

> Nurses do tend to get a bit more cynical as they get used to the job, as they feel more at home. So it is good to have someone more fresh. They are very good at talking to the patients and take a lot of time perhaps because they are not so aware of what is to be done.

Or:

> Too often we just well, we get into a rut of doing something and we just continue to do it because it has to be done and that's the way. Then you get the first-years and they are not so rushed and stressed as you are, and they don't have the responsibility and that allows them to step back a bit and ask 'why is it done like that?'

Another student described the 'uncanny way of getting to know your patients, which you seem to lose. You don't know half the technology which is going on around you. You are unaware of the necessity for speed to get all the jobs done. I used to often get shouted at, well sort of reminded that I had umpteen things to do when I was sitting there talking to patients'.

The first-year students were described in this way because they were still close enough to the beginning of their training to go beyond the medical labels to see the person behind the disease and to see talking to patients in the absence of technical knowledge as a central part of their work. Note how in Chapter 5 'talking' was seen as something to do after the 'real' work had been completed, except for a student at the beginning of training. Similarly, first-year students were 'not so aware' of what else had to be done (besides talking) and would be 'shouted at' or 'reminded' that they had 'umpteen [other] things to do', the 'real' work of bed-baths or tidying the sluice or linen cupboard.

These descriptions of the way in which students change are reminiscent of their changing perspectives on how they valued the content of nursing knowledge and practice. In Chapter 3 students shifted their views from seeing nursing as 'basics' and 'people' work to the absolute facts of 'diseases, drugs and therapy'. These perspectives are interconnected with their changing feelings about nursing and the loss of getting to know their patients, the acquisition of technical knowledge and feeling the need 'to get all the jobs done' under perceived pressure from trained staff.

The following account of a patient in pain, recounted by a student at the end of her first ward allocation, illustrates the 'uncanny way' a new nurse had of getting to know her patients, but who felt unable to persuade the trained staff to institute measures to relieve that pain. I asked her whether she could not have used the lunch-time report to make her observations and recommendations known to the trained staff, which was to increase the patient's analgesia. She was doubtful, feeling that her junior status prevented them taking her seriously, but also from seeing the person behind the pain, as a new entrant to nursing still could. Another explanation for the trained staff's reactions was that, drawing on the third-year accounts, they had 'got into a rut' of always doing things in the same way and feeling rushed and stressed to do the 'real' work, which prevented them from stepping back and asking 'why?' The student, still upset more than a week after leaving the ward, describes the incident from her point of view:

S. Joyce was in agony every time we moved her. If only they had given her something to kill the pain just an hour before we moved her, then it wouldn't be so hard lifting her. That's what she's going to be like for the rest of her life, every day, the same old pain.

Q. Was it not possible to give her painkillers?

S. You could tell the trained staff that the patient wants something, like the painkillers. I even wrote it in the kardex [nursing record]. But they [trained staff] gave the impression that you're not there to tell them what to do. They just thought she was a nuisance.

The student then went on to describe her reactions to what she saw as the trained staff's indifference.

I feel like I want to go out and change things already, like people in pain. What the hell! They're not going to get addicted. You just kill the pain.

I asked her what she meant about the patient 'getting addicted'. She said that she'd noticed that many nurses seemed reluctant to give patients too many painkillers because they believed they would get addicted to them.

Hayward (1975) reported similar findings in his study of nurses' management of patients' pain, and it is likely the student recalled the research from a recent class. In Joyce's case, the student believed the trained staff had 'overlooked' the need for pain control because they had not fully understood the extent of her pain.

> S. It would have been possible to give her painkillers but they just overlooked it. They just thought she was sitting there normally. Well she was but they didn't realise that every time we moved her she was in terrible pain.
>
> Q. How did you know?
>
> S. Well, we used to take her out of the ward in a wheelchair with her legs down and she was really shaking and I said 'Listen, I'll put the leg rest on, that'll be better' and after that we started using it. Nobody seemed to give her painkillers. She was on a lot of tablets, but I don't think they were painkillers. I think the doctors tend to be reluctant about painkillers anyway. It's like curing them without a cure. They think they're going to go downhill. She had Paget's disease which is difficult to cure.

This was perhaps an example of 'assembly line care of the sick' in which, as suggested by the student in Chapter 4, if the patient did not conform to the 'doctor's sort of norm' i.e. someone who could be 'cured' then they were at 'a loss what to do'. If the ward sisters also subscribed to a similar view of the work then the students were left on their own to deal best with their own preferences and priorities, especially at the beginning of training when they did not have any yardsticks by which to judge the alternatives.

In the recent study the target-driven health service provides a different type of yardstick which reinforces the notion of the 'assembly line care of the sick' to which students and staff alike are subject and the subsequent way in which work is organized may reduce perceived and actual opportunities to invest in patients in a personal way. However, as noted in Chapter 5, one important change that has taken place since the first study was reported has been the development of a range of specialist nurses including pain experts. It is likely that if ward staff in 2007 had been faced with a similar situation in which a patient like Miss Roberts had been in such agony they would have called on a specialist nurse to assist them to manage her pain.[1]

In 1984, however I was able to observe many examples of first-year students investing in patients in a personal way and making a significant contribution to their care. When, for example, students were given some choice over the patients allocated to their care, the first-years, and particularly those on their first ward, chose to care for the same patient, day after day. The first-ward students were more likely than any other group to ensure continuity of care for certain patients. Often these patients were the elderly, chronically sick and physically handicapped, like Joyce described above. Others included Bridget and Miss Roberts in Chapter 6.

The first-ward students, on the other hand, derived security from looking after the same patients over a period of time and consequently got to know them personally. But as the incidents of Joyce and others described elsewhere show, the students' junior status militated against the trained staff recognizing their insights and supporting their care. The other problem was that if their insights were not recognized and validated as 'work', the first-year students were not always able to respond therapeutically to their patients' emotional, and in the following case recounted by a tutor, physical needs.

A student described an incident where 'this patient was vomiting and was therefore unable to go home. And the first ward nurse simply couldn't cope with that. All she could say was "It'll be all right" over and over again'.

The first-ward nurse wanted to be with the patient and comfort her both because she was vomiting and also because of her disappointment at being unable to go home. Her lack of experience in coping with a vomiting patient apparently robbed her of her usual repertoire of reassuring words.

But there was also Miss Roberts' case, described in Chapter 6, where because Rachel, the first-year student, had got to know her over time she was able to give her loving care during her death agony. The staff nurse's sensitive care of both Rachel and Miss Roberts enabled her to do this.

During the second year, the students were allocated to specialist placements. They were often supernumerary, and they derived support not only from the trained staff but also from each other. It was during the second year that they were allocated to the psychiatric wards. As I described in Chapter 4, how these wards were explicitly geared towards communication and interpersonal skills, and provided the means by which the students learnt to do emotional labour. But they were quickly propelled back into the heady world of the acute general hospital where the predominant management styles packaged both them and their patients and gave them little opportunity to put these skills into practice.[2]

Students in the second study still experienced these culture shocks when moving between acute and community placements but rather than being concentrated in their second year, they were just as likely to occur at any stage during their three-year programme.

One student elaborated further:

We've been out of (hospital) practice for a year during our second year and it felt very strange coming back.

The result was that the student felt 'deskilled'. This phenomenon of placement sequence whereby students felt deskilled if their most recent placements had been spent in the community rather than acute care was described in Chapter 4 and was also apparent in the first study whereby acute medical and surgical care was seen as the cornerstone experience of the adult nursing student. However, in the second study 'the blues time' did not emerge as a phenomenon although as students continue to face particular challenges in their third year as they near the end of their training.

Third-year students: 'the blues time'

In 1984, the third and last year of training was difficult for students in that they were expected to be able to perform certain tasks by certain stages in their training, irrespective of actual experience, culminating in the ultimate emotional labour of them all described in Chapter 6: managing death and dying. The third years also felt that juniors got all the 'psychological support' whereas they were expected to 'cope on their own'.

The beginning of the third year was particularly difficult when students put on their red belt, the symbol of their seniority, for the first time. 'People (staff, patients, other students) just look at the belt', one student said 'and fail to realise the difference between someone just at the beginning of their third year or about to take their state finals'. They felt very unconfident to be back in the general wards after nearly a year of specialities where they were not the principal workforce. In 2010 the standard uniforms of white or blue tunic and navy blue trousers for all but the most senior nurses homogenized the nursing workforce. In some trusts nurses and health care assistants were distinguished by grade according to the colour of shoulder epaulettes, which they did not always wear and in any case were less distinctive than the different coloured belts.

In 1984, a number of students were feeling disillusioned, unhappy and considering leaving nursing at the beginning of their third year. One student grappling with this decision said:

> When I went through the stage of being generally fed up and talked to my friends, you'd be amazed! Some of them said it before I did. But according to one of the tutors it always happens at this stage of training. She called it the 'blues time' because she said 'It's recognised that people are disillusioned and fed up at this stage of nursing'.

The categorization of extreme feelings in this way 'normalized' them at risk of devaluing the personal difficulties that the student was going through. For this student, it was talking to other students rather than to the tutor which swayed her decision to stay in nursing. She said:

> When I spoke to some of my friends, I found that it's not just me. It's the place, the job. That's quite an exciting thing to discover that it's not just me.

Remember, too, the student in Chapter 4 who was allocated at the beginning of her third year to an oncology ward in the wake of her mother's death from cancer. The student felt very distressed by the experience, but neither did she feel she was able to tell anybody about her situation. So she just put up with feeling frustrated by patients who wouldn't help themselves and staff who appeared unsympathetic.

Amid all these feelings and life events, students had to prepare for their state final examinations. This period of training was also categorized by the tutors as a phase when students were described as suffering from 'tunnel vision' because they had one aim in the last months of training: to study as hard as they could in response to the prescriptive and formulaic format of their final examinations.

Reflections for the 2000s

The third year of training is still a difficult time for contemporary student nurses and during fieldwork they described feeling anxious and unprepared to operate as qualified nurses as they approached the completion of their programme.

The intuitive and holistic way that students were seen to operate in the first study as they progressed from first through to third year was not so apparent in the second study. As I described in previous chapters, students saw their clinical learning divided between personal care and technical tasks which were undertaken by designated members of the workforce namely health care assistants (HCAs) and registered nurses. This way of organizing the workforce on the one hand and the formal requirements of their academic programme on the other led to tailorized forms of learning. Awareness of being a first year or a third year student no longer seemed to form quite so explicit a part of the wider experience of being a student nurse but a discrete experience, placement by placement, rather than year on year. Another background factor was that many students had been HCAs either prior to beginning their formal programme and/or as a way of supplementing their bursaries. It is possible that this experience contributed to them not wanting to take on what was perceived as HCA work in lieu of learning technical nursing.

Personal emotion work

The questionnaire findings from the original study presented in Chapter 4 show that students felt comparatively high levels of anxiety and stress associated with feelings they were not generally expected either to feel or express, as in 'When the feelings don't fit'. The feeling rules of the City Hospital training were such that students undertook emotion work to suppress their feelings in public.

Students told me about the traumas of starting out on their training, the upheaval of leaving home and taking six months to settle down.

One student said:

I don't think I learnt much in my first six months as I was *frightened* ... I don't remember a great deal about it .... I think it was because I was *all tensed up*, really.

Being thrown in at the deep end

A common fear among students in the first study was that they would be 'thrown in at the deep end'. This meant they were fearful of the unknown, such as going to a ward for the first time with nobody to orientate them. I remember an occasion when working as a participant observer, a brand new first-warder arrived on the ward. The ward was very busy and short-staffed because one of the trained nurses was 'off sick'. The student was frequently left alone with patients, as the third-year student who was supposed to orientate her kept unavoidably rushing off with other patients to the operating theatres. Because I was supernumerary and able to fit in around the other nurses, I worked in place of the third-year student, planning and giving patient care with the first-warder. It is impossible to predict what the outcome would have been if I hadn't been on the ward that morning (I wasn't counted on the off duty rota), but there is a good chance that if I hadn't, the student would have felt she had been 'thrown in at the deep end' although she still felt relatively overwhelmed at the end of the morning's work.

Students in 2007 found themselves in comparable situations and also gave examples of undertaking emotion work associated with being thrown in at the deep end on account of insufficient guidance from mentors on the one hand or because they felt they lacked the necessary clinical skills expected of them at specific stages of their training on the other.

One student elaborated further explaining that one problem for her was the qualified staff's changing expectations that failed to take account of her learning needs. She said:

Sometimes I feel that too much is expected of me. I've found myself running a team and 10 patients and being expected to delegate and run the ward. Although this is what it's going to be like once I'm qualified I would have liked to have built up from five to 10 patients instead of being thrown into the deep end. I constantly have to ask for supervision, as it doesn't seem to be seen as a requirement by the trained staff.

Another student felt she had been thrown in at the deep end because 'the unit was so busy and staff over worked'. She suggested that mentors, being clear with students about their expectations as well as giving regular constructive feedback about their progress, would help to alleviate this feeling.

The consequences of inadequate mentoring were apparent in the following student account of 'feeling out of her depth':

Every experience is valuable, good and bad, you can learn from both, but for me I guess any situation when I am made to feel out of my depth and then guilty for not knowing the answer is not a good way to learn and undermines my confidence. This happened with my last mentor which is why I found it difficult to get on with her. I found her aggressive in the way she spoke and she made me feel very uncomfortable. As a result I became nervous and then I couldn't concentrate on what she was saying for fear she would suddenly put me on the spot. My co-mentors were the opposite and encouraged me to speak out and say what I thought and they didn't make me feel stupid if I was wrong. I felt confident at the beginning of my training but now as I progress I feel less and less confident which I find very worrying. Surely it should be building my confidence?

Another student felt that being treated as a member of the ward staff was 'good for learning'. But when the staff were 'so busy' she also felt as if she had been 'thrown in at the deep end'.

Yet another student wanted 'to be shown the ropes' in order 'to then gain confidence'. But a lack of sufficient mentors on the ward made her feel that:

I had to always be pushing for help. I found it stressful that I was feeling my way in the dark. I felt like I was thrown in at the deep end with inadequate support.

Another student felt she was 'in the dark' because of an interaction between stage of training (first year) and speciality (busy surgical ward) with its rapid pace of change. She said:

As a first year student I found it difficult to keep up with the changes happening on the busy ward: changes with patient's conditions and changes in nursing care. I was not always informed about the changes especially after doctors' rounds which made me feel like I was in the dark (cf. Melia 1984). It also made me feel like an outsider and caused me some stress and anxiety. Because students were expected to take part in the work load especially in the mornings, it made it difficult to learn new things. I felt stress because I was worried about my learning. Opportunities were there, but I could not go and learn, because I was busy delivering basic care.

The student shared the view of many of her peers that 'delivering basic care' was an obstacle rather than integral to learning and nursing work.

One third year student described the interaction between seniority and a 'new' speciality such as Accident and Emergency (A&E) which made her feel out of her depth:

A&E was a very different experience from my other ward placements and although I enjoyed the placement, I felt a little out of my depth at times. There are high expectations for third year students but the critical care placements are very much new territory for us.

Another student described a similar reaction to the specialist work of the health visitor which she experienced as part of her community nursing placement:

I felt out of my depth sometimes as I am doing the Adult program and my placement was with a health visitor. I don't have children myself and felt that I knew very little about parenthood, infants and young children. These areas are very specific to health visitors/midwives and although we had been educated in the role of these nurses, we had not been educated in the health issues which these professionals give advice and assistance for.

Another contributing factor as to why students in the 2000s felt out of their depth was frequently attributed to length of placement. Many placements were shorter than the standard eight weeks of the first study. As one student explained:

Sadly this placement is only for four weeks and I feel that I would benefit from a longer placement here.

The combination of pressure of the workload and inadequate support led to another student feeling out of her depth because she did not 'know or understand what was required of me'.

Students also saw that being 'out of their depth' could be indicative of being 'encouraged to try new things' and therefore a 'natural' reaction.

On my last placement I felt out of my depth, but this is only natural as I was encouraged to try new things, unlike some of my other placements where I was not encouraged to really learn at all.

Such feelings could be countered by a well-planned 'training environment' as the following student explained:

This training environment has been well planned and thought out. Because it is within SHDU (Surgical High Dependency Unit) the first few days were a huge learning curve and I did feel out of my depth initially. However the staff have been very supportive and because I have been able to consolidate what I have learnt, I am feeling more confident and I want to push my learning further.

Another student was helped to deal with a 'very stressful environment' by 'friendly staff':

As I was placed on AICU (Acute Intensive Care Unit) it was a very stressful environment because of the specialized area of care that was being given. Most patients we were caring for were critical and many died, but I feel the staff made sure that as students we got the support we needed and I rarely felt stressed as I was made to feel relaxed in the area I was working in through the support from the friendly staff.

Other positive learning experiences were described in relation to 'working alongside' a nurse in caring for a patient who was critically ill:

On the days when I was working alongside a nurse with a more critical patient, I could watch procedures such as tracheotomy care, talk through them and then perform them under supervision the next time. I find this the best way to learn.

Another student found her critical care module to be invaluable in dealing with deteriorating patients:

The ward on which I worked had a four bedded HDU (High Dependency Unit); this gave me invaluable experience in dealing with deteriorating patients. I was taught the evidence base behind escalating care for such patients. I also gained valuable experience in basic nursing care for critically ill patients, particularly in considering the finer details of care and in anticipating the patient's needs and being prepared for this.

And yet another student said:

The critical care aspect of the placement allowed me to think on my feet and provide care quickly.

In the first study, students were particularly apprehensive of night duties when staffing levels could be low and patients very sick, like the night I spent on Mr Brown's ward described in Chapter 6. They were particularly fearful of their first set of night duty after only six months' training. One student told me how she had spent her first holiday worrying about 'going on nights'. In the recent study night duty was not so much an issue for students as they were only expected to be part of the night duty rota at the end of their third year and under supervision.

Other students in the first study, even when they were well into their third year, experienced the first few weeks of a new allocation as a very anxious time. One student told me: 'I don't know if anyone really appreciates how anxious you are starting a new ward'. Another student told me that she found it easier to slip into the ward routine as a third-year: 'It used to sometimes take me three or four weeks, especially if there was a difficult staff relationship. Now I feel quite relaxed after about two weeks'. Another third-year student appeared 'really down' during her first few days on the ward according to a first-year, but 'really changed' after she had settled down. I was working as a participant observer on the same ward at the time and also noticed how the third-year student visibly relaxed and smiled more after a week or so. I remember her on her first morning coming up to me and asking rather apologetically (third-year students were supposed to know everything) if I could show her how a catheter leg bag worked, never having seen that particular type of appliance before.

Trained staff in the 1980s also saw the contribution of 'kind and quiet' third-years who 'change the atmosphere' of the ward. The contribution made by students to the learning environment, particularly the 'mature' students, who showed great awareness of the need to support their mentors was also apparent in the second study as described in Chapter 5. There was the student who 'did training in previous jobs' that allowed her to put herself in the mentor's shoes and to recognize there might be times when the demands of patient care required her to 'take a step back' to let the mentor 'have that space'. Another third year student realized there may be times when the focus could not be on the student but had to be on the patient. Students' recognition of the need to be conscious and aware of the needs of mentors and patients were examples of personal emotion work on their part.

The weight of the nursing hierarchy in dictating students' roles and relationships was particularly evident in the 1980s and suggested by the following statement, made by a student just beginning her third ward allocation. This was the first time in her training that she had had students junior to herself. She said:

It's strange when you've actually got someone turning round and asking you something. You're not quite the bottom of the dirt pile anymore.

Feeling that they were at the bottom of a dirt pile explains the helplessness and frustration that juniors felt in influencing patients' care without the support of their seniors.

In the first study one way students learnt to appear confident was through their assessments which also reinforced their roles and relationships at different stages of their trajectory, so that they felt able to support other students.

Third-year students recognized that they were important to the juniors because:

We aren't quite so detached as the trained staff. You feel more like the first-years do.

Another student said:

You forget how as a first-year you are frightened of approaching anybody more senior than you.

This observation is illustrated by the following incident, recounted by a senior third-year student who took on the responsibility for having a word with a first-year student who was too frightened to address the ward sister directly.

Sister was standing next to me during the drug round and a first-year student came up to me and said 'Could you tell sister that Mr Green's temperature has gone up?' Well [laughing] Sister, she just died! She said 'I think she's a bit scared to talk to me don't you?' so I thought, 'I had better have a word and say "well, sister won't bite you!"'. But then there must be some kind of awe still for the first-years. I mean I remember feeling frightened of the sister when I first started training, but you forget quite easily.

This incident illustrates the power of the hierarchy in provoking feelings of fear in a student (at the bottom of the dirt pile) to the extent that she felt unable to address the ward sister face to face, but had to go through an intermediary. It also illustrates the responsibility the third-year student felt to act as an intermediary on behalf of the junior student.

But there was also the perspective that you had to do emotion work on yourself in order to deal with the hierarchy and your fear of it. One student told me:

I found that it's up to you to brave the initial fear of a trained staff uniform and ask questions. If that staff member remembers what it's like to be a first-year nurse then your individuality is preserved.

These hierarchical relationships and differentiation between first and third-year students did not seem so explicit in the later study. Rather these relationships needed to be explored in relation to the division of labour that has driven a wedge between the personal care undertaken by the HCAs and the technical work of the qualified nurse. Students' constant reference to not wanting to do what they perceived to be 'health care assistant work' suggests that HCAs as a group may be seen to be at the bottom of the 'dirt pile' of the contemporary division of labour. As Johnson et al. (2004) cited in Chapter 1 suggest, even in a prestigious speciality such as critical care, the main aspiration of the HCA role was to 'relieve qualified nurses from routine', which reinforces the stereotype of personal care as lower status work.

Caring factors

What then were the factors in 1984 that influenced the students' caring styles and capacity during their three-year trajectory and their choice of future emotional styles?

Ward management styles: recognizing or repressing individuality

In Chapter 5 ward sisters' management styles were characterized according to whether they managed their wards through hierarchy and tasks as part of the 'assembly line care of the sick' or by 'nurturing' people. Students found themselves caught between these competing management styles as they moved from ward to ward. During any one allocation, the extent to which a sister's ward management style recognized or repressed a student's individuality (i.e. a style that nurtured people or managed tasks) emerged as an important factor in the caring trajectory. The importance of recognizing a student's individuality has already been suggested by the student's comment above, who describes the importance of the trained staff remembering 'what it's like to be a first-year'. It is more likely that students are able to approach ward sisters who are committed to people, rather than hierarchy and tasks, and that these sisters will remember their own feelings as junior nurses.

The importance of management styles in recognizing or repressing a student's individuality were described by a nurse tutor in the following way:

> Every ward operates in its own way. It's a culture shock. Some wards encourage the students as individuals and others repress it. It varies with the individual as to what happens when they go to the ward.

Every eight weeks the students were required to adjust their preferences and priorities to individual styles of management that either encouraged or repressed their individuality.

But the tutor also described how different students perceived their ward experiences differently. She said: 'It's fascinating to see their reactions, because you can have two people sitting there and you don't know they're talking about the same ward'. When I asked the tutor why she thought students reacted so differently, she said: 'It's their personality, expectations, what they've heard on the grapevine and whether the individual style of management suits them'.

Similar factors were in play in the recent study. Presently, the mentor holds the key to the 'caring' side described by a link lecturer in Chapter 5 as 'the humanistic approach' towards students. The development of a successful mentoring relationship was shown to be essential to student nurse learning and dependent on the staff having a welcoming attitude to them, not seeing them as a pair of hands and offering them clear learning opportunities.

And from a student's perspective:

> I thoroughly enjoyed this placement and learned a lot about individuals and how different patients react to a situation. I also saw that the nurses were genuinely interested in the patients they cared for and were willing to listen to their problems or explain things to them. This ward also had a much more relaxed atmosphere, something I had not seen on other placements, which was also commented on by patients. This is a good ward to learn both the basics of patient care such as rapport and communication but also to learn in depth about the disease processes of different cancers and the types of treatment given to either treat the disease or its symptoms.

The fact that 'a relaxed atmosphere' on the ward seemed as if it might be unusual is substantiated by other students who frequently commented on the lack of an emotionally caring style on many wards so that they neither felt welcome nor a member of the ward team. But on a ward where staff were 'genuinely interested in patients' and 'willing to listen' the student was able to recognize and learn about the importance of rapport and communication with patients and not just about disease processes and treatment.

There were a number of resonances with the first study in this student's comment. The first was the recognition of the relaxed ward atmosphere by both students and patients and the inference that this was important for both caring and learning. The second was the connection between good communication and rapport on a cancer ward where emotional care was legitimated and students also reported learning technical skills.

It has already been noted that supernumerary status has since changed the students' learning experiences and heightened awareness of their need to learn as well as work and that they were more likely to have a positive experience when 'the number of staff was adequate for the workload'. As one student advised it was then possible to:

> Shadow one nurse all shift and learn and build up a good working relationship – which helps to makes students feel as if they are working as part of a team!

There was also the third year student quoted in Chapter 5 who described her mentor who was also the ward manager as 'brilliant,' 'quite strict' and respected by all, who encouraged her to think for herself.

These comments confirm the findings that resources, in particular a workforce adequate for the workload and positive relationships with trained staff are important to create an environment that is conducive to learning and caring. They also connect with the findings in the first study in which I considered the mechanisms and motivations that brought trained staff and students together at different stages of their trajectory in order to see how the students' own caring styles and capacity might be either reinforced or discouraged by particular management styles over time. Because of their experiences on particular wards at particular times, students began to form their own preferences and priorities for their future work and to decide which 'style of management suits'.

In the first study, the sisters and staff nurses who had chosen to work together formed a cohesive group which supported a particular philosophy and style. Students, on the other hand, had little say over their ward placements and were allocated for an eight-week period to fulfil their training requirements and the staffing needs of the hospital.

Junior students were conscious that the ward hierarchy made them 'vulnerable' and 'on the side of the patient'. They were more likely to start out seeing things from the patient's rather than the staff's perspective. The staff nurses might regard patients as 'awkward' and 'up to their old tricks' rather than looking for reasons for their behaviour. Students were less willing to accept labels and stereotypes, but they also found difficulty in resisting the opinions of their hierarchical superiors as the 'experts'. Even when students disagreed with the ward staff's opinions on patients and their care, hierarchical management styles prevented them from either offering alternative perspectives or feeling they could offer such alternatives. The first-year student who cared for Joyce, described at the beginning of this chapter, offers one such example. Although she had found her own ways of relieving Joyce's pain, she also felt unable to challenge the staff's view of Joyce as 'a nuisance'.

The issue of hierarchy as a mechanism for shaping emotional labour for more senior students also arises from the critical incident from the first study described in Chapter 3. The student, commenting on the incident, observed that her fellow student, also a third-year, 'knew she didn't do what she should have done as a nurse' by convincing a distraught relative to take her psychiatrically disturbed brother home because the medical and trained staff wanted him out of their ward. The pressures put on the student to conform to the wishes of those higher up in the hierarchy made it very difficult for her to maintain her own person-orientated perspective, and she found herself undertaking emotional labour to satisfy the wishes of those in authority rather than to do 'what she should have done' which was to insist that the patient stayed in hospital.[3]

Sister Ronda would not accept labels and stereotypes and used the ward handover report to explore why students thought patients were behaving in certain ways. She also sought students' opinions and perceptions on patients and their care.

There were still some students, particularly the third-years who had been exposed to task-orientated nursing and hierarchically managed wards and were resistant to Sister Ronda's preferences and priorities, such as the student who found that patient allocation 'went too far'.

I observed another incident when a third-year student disagreed with Sister's decision not to sedate a patient with dementia during the day. The patient was quite noisy and tried to get up from her chair to stagger unsteadily around the ward. The student objected on three counts. The patient was disruptive to other patients; she might fall and hurt herself; and she was more difficult to nurse in that she had to be interacted with. This third consideration was the sister's intention, since she wanted the students to interact with the patient in order to make her feel safe and cared for rather than drugged and remote. The third-year student would fume in the sluice, feeling that she had 'better' things to do. She was having to do emotional labour (suppress feelings in private) in order to present her calm City nurse exterior to the external world of the ward. The difference between Sister Ronda and many other sisters was that she would listen to the student's point of view. For the student however, this did not help as she did not agree with the sister's preferences and priorities, having now formed her own. She was looking forward to the end of her training, when she hoped to become a staff nurse on a surgical ward where the work was organized in a more task-orientated and hierarchical way.

Now students are more likely to be exposed to target-driven cultures so are not familiar with patient allocation as a way of organizing the work. They also see their roles at different stages of their training according to what people do rather than a holistic view of nursing. The end result is similar to their predecessors with their overriding ambition being to undertake technical nursing tasks such as the drug rounds, aseptic dressings, catheterization and inserting naso-gastric tubes and will only do the personal care work when HCAs are not available or until the opportunity to do 'real nursing work' becomes available. This shift to a workforce model of nursing delivery, reinforced by the target driven culture of the NHS is more in line with 'the assembly line care of the sick' described in the first study. They reach the end of their training feeling unprepared and inadequate for the technical and management roles they are expected to fulfil as qualified nurses. However they also have other role models such as clinical nurse specialists and practitioners to whom to aspire. The students are most likely to encounter nursing specialists during their 'spokes' experiences associated with a 'hub' speciality. In Chapter 5, for example, one student spoke enthusiastically of her time with the tissue viability specialist whom she recognized as 'great at what she did' in an 'essential' speciality.

In Chapter 5 I describe how aspects of ward handover and patient allocation have changed. To some extent this change relates to the introduction of supernumerary status. In order to be an effective learner, student nurses now have to negotiate their position within the ward team and with their mentor. They do this by finding out how clinical staff in each placement view supernumerary status and act according to those expectations. When the first study took place, expectation by ward staff was very important to the students. It continues to be so but the expectations are different and relate to students' changed status as supernumerary rather than paid frontline workers and the dissonance expressed by trained staff as to how students used to be and how they are now. The relationship between first and third-year students and their clear progression through different stages of their trajectory have changed so that they are no longer apprentices and their learning outcomes define their work rather than their year of training.

Allocation of the workload by ward managers to meet students' learning needs was variable. On one ward the ward manager organized the work by asking students what they wanted to do, whether their mentors were on duty and was aware that a third year student had a drugs assessment coming up. On another ward the allocation of students to mentors during handover was not so well organized, and it became apparent that one student took the initiative to allocate her own and her fellow student's work as Helen's field notes indicate:

> When the ward manager came out of the office she had two staff nurses, then two students trailing behind; the allocation had already been done. Students looked hesitant but then started to hand out breakfasts. Later during coffee a third year student expressed anger about what had happened at the start of the shift in which she had had to take stock and assess the workload so that she could take account of her learning needs.

The student explained:

> The staff nurses were already busy on the phone so we had to do the work, decide what to do. No-one supervises you.

A theme to emerge from these observations was that the contemporary student needs to be an active learner who can successfully negotiate with the ward staff to meet their learning objectives, while becoming an integrated member of the ward team. Such potentially complex negotiations require the emotional qualities of confidence and determination. Put another way students may need to use their emotional labour to develop emotional intelligence[4] in order to survive and thrive in the target and outcome-orientated environment of the 2000s.

Ward management styles: recognizing the student's learning role

Recognition of the student's learning role was a factor associated with management styles that helped students to feel that they were being recognized as individuals. In the first study third-year students warned me when I distributed the ward learning environment questionnaires that I could expect lower scores because they felt less positive than the first-years about their training. When I analysed the questionnaire scores I did indeed find that the first-year students' average ratings for the ward learning environment were generally higher than later in training (see: Companion website, Appendix E, Tables E12-E15, Smith 1992). I put this down to the cynicism and disillusion that the third-years complained of and their resentment at being used as 'pairs of hands'.

Differences between first and third years were less easy to detect in the 2007 survey partly because of the design of the survey but also because as the qualitative data suggested, the issue of being used as a 'pair of hands' cropped up throughout the students' three-year experience. Further analysis of the open-ended survey comments by student year revealed that the contemporary student still favours acute technical specialities over and above older peoples' care and that the first year continues to be seen as the most appropriate stage of training to be placed in a care home or older people's ward.

I wanted to further investigate the earlier finding that when ward sisters recognised the students' learning role they felt valued and better equipped to care for patients irrespective of speciality or year of training. Were similar relationships still apparent in the learning environment of the 2000s? The findings presented in Chapter 5 suggest that this is still the case but articulated through the mentor who may not necessarily be the ward manager or ward sister.

In 1984, Sister Edale, for example, whose ward got top scores, clearly articulated the relationship between teaching students and ensuring patients got good care.

One student explained the importance of a management style that also recognized the student's learning role in the following way:

> When you go to a ward the extent to which you *enjoy* the experience, isn't related to the sort of nursing you are doing [i.e. the ward speciality]. It's much more what the atmosphere of the ward is like and *who you are working with*. I think where there is a lot of input from ward staff and they want to teach you, you get a lot more from it and you're *happier* about nursing the patients because you've got more information.

This student articulates the relationship between the trained staff's express commitment to teaching as part of creating the 'caring' atmosphere, the importance of good working relations and the generation of positive feelings: enjoyment and happiness associated with having more information about nursing the patients. I am inferring that a student who enjoys a clinical placement and feels happier is less likely to feel stress and anxiety, which is confirmed by findings presented in Chapter 5.

Personal support

In 1984, the recognition of the student learning role was one important way in which students felt supported. But, in general, they were incredulous at the lack of support they got throughout their training from either their teachers or their ward sisters. They felt that there was no one person who was there for them as an individual. It is little wonder that they talked about becoming cynical in the so-called caring profession that didn't demonstrate any care of its most junior and largest group of carers. One student admitted that 'if you wanted support the tutors would give it, but because there's no opportunity to build up a relationship with them, they're like strangers'. The student was emphasizing the importance she attached to good personal relationships, which depended on getting to know someone.

One student said:

> Third-years support first-years on some wards but everyone needs it, as well as reassurance. The third-years get cross at not getting support. Third-years are just expected to cope.

Sister Windermere played a vital role in supporting a third-year student going through the so-called blues time. She noticed how unhappy she looked while allocated to her ward. She called the student into her office during a quiet period on the evening shift in order to find out the cause of her unhappiness. She was able to talk her through some of her difficulties and discouraged her from leaving nursing at that late stage in her training. The student concluded that:

> I was going through a period of wanting to leave nursing whilst I was on Windermere ward, but sister recognised this and was very supportive through a difficult period.

If students felt psychologically supported throughout their training then they were more likely to sustain caring styles and capacities that recognized and valued emotional labour as part of their work. What emerged in the first study was the importance of the third-year students in the production and reproduction of emotional labour, not only in relation to the patients and the smooth running of the ward, but principally in supporting the junior students.

In the later study, questionnaire and fieldwork findings showed that the mentor emerged as key to recognizing the student's learning role. The ward manager or sister was not necessarily the individual that developed that direct relationship with the student but they were key in as much as they created the environment for positive student mentoring and team working. Although students could be an important support to each other they needed to adopt the role of active learner, able to negotiate complex relationships with a diverse nursing workforce from health care assistants to ward managers and the interface between academic study and practice.

The caring-learning relationship and emotional labour

The complexity of the caring-learning relationships in which a student finds herself on her trajectory are graphically expressed by a third-year student in the 1984 study:

> In nursing you have got so many relationships to form with people who you have never met before, who you probably don't like, you may not like out of work, under circumstances that are tremendously difficult. Often the relationships are short and sharp

with hierarchy and authority and discipline somewhere mixed up into them, the learning situation as well.

This student was saying many things of relevance to the emotional labour analysis. Firstly, she drew attention to the central issue of personal relationships in nursing. Many times during this and previous chapters the centrality of relationships in caring and feeling cared for have been highlighted. Often nurses found themselves working with people they did not like (both patients and other nurses), but felt they had to suppress these feelings. Often the relationships were short and sharp, because students constantly changed wards and most patients were 'just passing through'. The shift systems were such that contact between staff, students and patients tended to be fragmented and to lack continuity, even in the nursing process era.

Attention is also drawn to the importance of hierarchy, authority and discipline in shaping these relationships. As seen above certain management styles and the assessment system could repress rather than encourage a student in her efforts to sustain an individual commitment to caring. It is possible that if a student is repressed too often for too long, coupled with the need to suppress her own personal feelings, it is more likely that she will choose hierarchical relationships, labelling and stereotypes as the preferred form of emotional labour by the end of her trajectory.

If we examine from the point of view of the trajectory, we begin to see that if students are constantly exposed to 'circumstances that are tremendously difficult', which I interpret as a lack of caring factors, they will either choose to leave or to develop styles to protect their emotions. The issue remains pertinent to the current study in which mature students and the life experiences they bring to their understanding of the caring trajectory is a new dimension to consider.

Emotional labour: styles and strategies

The 1980s

In the first study, nurses developed strategies to deal with extreme feelings. These included various 'distancing' strategies such as developing a 'seen it all before attitude' which made it easier to label patients and their behaviour. Thus by slotting patients into convenient categories such as 'difficult', 'awkward', 'a pain' or 'a nuisance', and projecting images and assumptions upon them associated with their gender, class and race, as described in Chapter 4, nurses were able to 'objectify' them and their symptoms.

The students' accounts in Chapter 6 suggested that repeated confrontation with death and laying people out on an oncology ward made even them 'blasé', after only an eight-week allocation. The students reasoned that prolonged exposure to continual death and dying made the permanent staff appear 'hard' in an attempt to distance themselves from their feelings, in a reverse form of emotional labour. When students returned from their days off wanting to find out what had happened to the patients they had cared for on night duty, they found that 'the trained staff just didn't want to know'. Or the staff nurse who had to walk away from Mr Lawrence because she found his crying every time she talked to him too difficult to cope with. On many wards, the trained staff physically removed themselves from patient and even student contact by going to their offices.

The way in which nursing was traditionally organized around tasks reduced close nurse-patient encounter and reduced anxiety.[5] Even though the nursing process had been introduced to encourage nurses to care for patients rather than to carry out tasks, most ward sisters operated a system that allowed students some choice over the patients they cared for. With the exception of students at the beginning of training, they were likely to change their allocation daily, which permitted them to regulate their personal involvement with patients.

Evidence suggests that these strategies were developed during the caring trajectory if students were repeatedly exposed to a range of emotionally demanding experiences without the support of their hierarchical superiors. Joining 'the other side' in labelling and stereotyping patients was one way of reducing the conflict between their commitment to care and the prevailing ward philosophy and style.

Even a first-warder after only eight weeks on a ward told me: 'It's good to stop and think about how people feel, otherwise you treat them like objects'. Or consider a third-year student who said that:

> It is very hard to appreciate how patients actually feel about what is wrong with them unless you talk to them.

At this point I recall the haunting words of the first-year student who said: 'if people don't matter then you can't do nursing', a theme that returns again and again. A student nearing the end of her training also uttered similar words, but added a caveat. She said:

> I came into nursing to care for people. I expected to care for them in pain and when they were dying. What I didn't expect was that the system doesn't always let me do it in the way I want to.

Students were more likely to feel this way on wards where the sisters managed hierarchically and produced a negative emotional labour which made nurses feel frightened, anxious and stressed.

The divisiveness of the hierarchy was apparent in the way in which it separated the trained staff from the students and transformed them into pairs of hands for performing tasks rather than patient-centred care.

The formal content of student nurse training gave them little guidance on managing complex feelings or on offering a viable alternative to the biomedical base of nursing. They also received little personal support throughout their training from either teachers or ward sisters. But there were also many Sister Rondas, who showed that it is possible to maintain caring styles and capacity over time and to reproduce the nurse with 'the caring side' from one generation to the next. The principal variable was feeling cared for themselves and supported, which allowed the nurses to care more for each other and ultimately the patients. The recognition of nursing as people work was at the crux, which made emotional care visible and valued in both the form and content of their training.

First-year students invested in patients in a personal way and made a significant contribution to their care. When given the choice they often opted to care for patients on a daily basis. Many of these patients were often seen as 'only' requiring basic nursing and hence within the scope of a first-year student. As students progressed through their trajectory their expectations for nursing changed. They became more concerned to consolidate their technical and managerial skills, but were also expected to take on organizational and other responsibilities, irrespective of their previous experiences, by trained staff.

Third-year students underwent a stressful period known locally as the 'blues time'. It was during that period that a number of students grappled with the decision of whether to leave nursing or not.

Throughout their three-year programme nurses experienced a range of emotions associated with both their personal and training trajectory. They received little formal support and undertook emotional labour to conceal these feelings from the outside world.

The nursing hierarchy and the assessment system dictated students' roles and relationships. Third-year students were particularly important in their support of junior students and many of them undertook emotional labour to make them feel safe and cared for.

A number of caring factors were identified which influenced students' caring styles and capacities over time and their personal choice of future forms of emotional labour. Of critical importance was the ward sister's management style in encouraging or repressing students' individuality throughout the trajectory. The nursing hierarchy played an important role in shaping emotional labour and the students' capacity to care throughout their trajectory.

The recognition of the students' learning role by the ward sister was also identified as an important caring factor. Personal support given to students was *ad hoc* and depended on the ward sister's management style rather than teachers in the school of nursing.

Finally, the complexity of the caring–learning relationship is described, drawing on the analysis of a quote from a third-year student in which she describes the fragmentation of personal relationships between nurses and between nurses and patients. I speculate that if students' individuality and caring commitment is repressed too often and for too long during their three-year trajectory, coupled with the need to suppress their own personal feelings, then it is likely that they will chose hierarchical relations, stereotyping and labelling as preferred forms of emotional labour by the end of that trajectory.

Unless students were supported by their teachers and ward sisters, they developed styles and strategies which enabled them to distance themselves from patients to protect their own feelings in a reverse form of emotional labour.

But there were also ward sisters with management styles that showed that the critical variable which allowed nurses to maintain 'a caring side' and to reproduce it from one generation to the next was feeling cared for themselves. This required the recognition of nursing as predominantly people work which made emotional care visible and valued in both the form and content of their training.[6]

The 2000s

The current study revealed that students still complained of being used as 'pairs of hands', but they were just as likely to feel this way in their first year and throughout their training. The hierarchy continued to act divisively by separating them not only from the trained staff above them but from the HCAs below who had inherited the vital personal care work that first-year students in the first study had associated with being used as 'just a pair of hands'.

The formal content of nurse training was found to be highly regulated and prescribed, and students were required to satisfy their learning objectives at the end of each placement which could potentially constrain what they saw as learning and learning opportunities. Chapter 3 set out the contemporary prescription for learning as specified in the benchmarks, frameworks and code of conduct which consistently include communication, compassion, care and prioritization of patient need as essential nursing competences. But there was also a sense that the students took initiatives to negotiate their way as supernumerary learners to meet their learning outcomes but at the same time were aware of negotiating on behalf of their co-students. The mentoring relationship is at the core and 'mature' nursing students were able to bring their life experience to be supportive and collegiate towards their mentors and to negotiate their relationship which allowed them to both care for patients as well as facilitate their learning.

The student's learning trajectory is orchestrated by a highly prescriptive and regulated curriculum and mediated by the mentor who also holds the key to the 'caring' side of nursing, described in Chapter 5 as 'the humanistic approach'. This approach facilitates the development of a successful mentoring relationship that welcomed students and viewed them primarily as learners rather than a 'pair of hands'. In the same way as their predecessors needed to feel cared for in order to care for others, contemporary students had similar requirements. The recognition of the 'caring' side of nursing is becoming increasingly challenged by technically orientated learning objectives and mentors who have to manage a rapid patient throughput in the acute hospital setting as well as supporting student learning. The students no longer progress through an apprentice style trajectory learning tasks and skills appropriate to their year of training but are more bound by a hierarchy of skills associated with hierarchical roles within the nursing division of labour.

A number of important questions emerge from these findings which I shall explore in the final chapter. These questions relate to the role of the HCA in the wider health and social care context, the persistence of the stereotype that placements other than in acute settings are not valuable to learning, the way in which the mentor holds the key to the 'caring' side of nursing, the meaning of supernumerary status and being used as pairs of hands. Students' experience of mentoring was very variable and was also influenced by their outlook, experience and maturity. In particular students' role as active learners and negotiators of complex relationships may require them not only to undertake emotional labour but develop emotional intelligence in order to survive and thrive in the target and outcome-orientated environment of the 2000s. These questions and others are particularly pertinent as nursing moves towards all-graduate entry by 2013.

Conclusions

Readers of my first book experienced it as 'a voyage of discovery', a quest for understanding of what lay at the heart of nursing. Their experiences accurately reflect not only what the research was about, but how I went about it. I wanted to discover what learning to care meant to students in terms of both its content and process. The original chapters were written in the spirit of that discovery in order to draw conclusions on the meaning of care, its interpretation and transmission in ward and classroom and its effects on nurses and patients.

The second book is based on a different approach combining research, experience and policy changes. The first book was a direct outcome of my doctoral research which I lived and breathed for four years from 1984 to 1988 including one year of in-depth field work. The notion of emotional labour was introduced to the world of sociology in 1983 by Professor Arlie Hochschild, and I applied it to the world of nursing at about the same time. I later spent a further six months during 1990 converting the doctoral thesis into a popular book, which was published in 1992. In the intervening years, changes have taken place in the UK health and educational system which have impacted on student nurses' learning, and I was keen to follow up on my original emotional labour research. I was especially interested in nursing's move to higher education, the replacement of apprentice trainees by supernumerary students and the changes in nursing leadership and ward sister roles in the 'new' NHS (Smith and Gray, 2001a, 2001b; Allan et al. 2008a, 2008b). In this second book I have drawn on a number of studies to interrogate my original data to provide a window on the world of contemporary student nurses and nursing and to ask can nurses still care in the NHS of the twenty-first century? In this final chapter I revisit my original conclusions to consider that question.

Concepts of care and emotional labour

Care is a complex concept. In the 1980s, nursing leaders exhorted nurses to care, but their definitions were limited by their failure to take into account the emotional complexity of caring. Neither did they consider the way in which care is stereotyped as women's 'natural' work, as part of the gender division of labour nor the power relations between doctors (predominantly men) and nurses (predominantly women) within a health service which marginalized care as the little things.

In 2011, the power relations between the professions remain, although the gender stereotypes are not quite straightforward. While the percentage of men in nursing has stayed roughly the same at ten per cent, the percentages of women entering medicine has increased to over fifty per cent. Nursing remains a predominantly female occupational group and the hostile reaction to the announcement that it was to become a graduate-only profession was interpreted by some commentators as reflecting the public perception that academic study was not required for undertaking a job that was vocational and primarily concerned with caring and women's work.

Although care remains a contested issue, nurses and patients continue to describe it as the essential ingredient of the 'good' nurse. Care is associated with the emotional component of nursing which underpins both technical and physical activities. A key finding in my original research was that student nurses felt better able to care for patients when they felt cared for themselves by the trained ward staff and their teachers. Because care was such a marginalized activity and so conceptually ill defined, I wanted to draw on my data to re-define it. The accounts of caring from both students and patients suggested that 'caring' did not come naturally. Nurses had to work emotionally on themselves in order to appear to care, irrespective of how they personally felt about themselves, individual patients, their conditions and circumstances. They could also be taught to manage their feelings more effectively.

Students felt frustrated when the system prevented them from caring, a feeling compounded in the 2000s by the combined effects of the target-driven culture and clinical learning objectives to become technically competent nurses. Health care assistants (HCAs) rather than students were the primary givers of personal care while students aspired to being competent in the technical tasks of becoming a registered nurse which potentially prevented them from seeing holistic care as part of their learning trajectory. The competing demands on students to learn and care during their placements made them sometimes feel like they were in a 'hostile environment'. Students more than ever needed to feel cared for in the practice settings, described by one lecturer as the 'humanistic approach' where the 'little things' still mattered and students felt welcome and safe. The end result was that they felt able to both negotiate their learning as supernumerary learners but also their responsibility to patients.

In the first study the data analysis was inspired by Arlie Hochschild's (1983) definition of emotional labour. I did not start out with the notion of care as emotional labour, but my data led me to select an appropriate framework. I then put

Arlie's definition and analysis of emotional labour to the test each time I asked questions of my data. In this way I was able to assess its theoretical viability in the context of nursing. I was interested to find therefore that Nicky James (1986) had chosen to combine the two terms in her research, by referring to nursing the dying as 'carework'. The importance of defining care as work cannot be underestimated if this most essential ingredient of what nurses do is to be recognized and valued. But recognition and value are not enough. Care must be supported educationally and organizationally in the institutions where nurses work and learn and by the political and economic structures within society (Tronto 1987).

The management of feelings and the conceptual and operational devices available to recognize the role of emotions in both learning and caring have become more explicit over the years and the emotional labour literature has expanded its repertoire to include a variety of models and interdisciplinary approaches to encompass psychoanalysis and psychology as well as sociology. Emotional intelligence has also been presented as a way of understanding the broader dimensions of emotions by going beyond the feeling rules to recognize the diversity of human relationships and potentially competing expectations when working in complex organizations. Nurse education therefore needs to equip students at a very early stage to be emotionally competent if 'they are to be successful in their working environment' (Bellack 1999).

In the 2010s, one way in which care is recognized is through the language of compassion and is articulated as a key component of nursing and nurse education. For example, the requirement for a compassionate practitioner is explicit in the Nursing and Midwifery Council's current and new pre-registration curricula and standards which will inform the development of all future programmes. Two national projects (Cornwell and Goodrich 2009; www.napier.ac.uk/ccnews) provide approaches to defining and attaining the elusive but highly prized goal of compassionate care. There are also a variety of tools available such as the compassion index (Department of Health 2008) and 'emotional touch points' (Bate and Robert 2007, Dewar et al. 2010) to assist thinking about the processes and outcomes of care, reminiscent of my use of emotional labour as a conceptual device to understand how students learnt to care.

These compassionate care trends were pulled together by former Prime Minister Gordon Brown's commission on nursing and midwifery. Brown's commitment to compassion was evident in his address to the Royal College of Nursing Congress in 2009:

I think you judge a country and you judge the people of a country not by the size of their wallets but by the breadth of their compassion, by the depth of their generosity, by the width of their goodness and there is no profession that deserves the title of being the most compassionate profession than nursing today (Brown 2009, http://www.rcn.org.uk/newsevents/news/article/uk/ brown_and_cameron_address_delegates_in_historic_day_at_congress).

These words were spoken in the final stages of gathering evidence for the commissioners' report which reinforced the compassion agenda and further embedded it in the language of educational curricula and practice standards.

At the time of writing the first book the gendered nature of nursing work and the perpetuation and predominance of the Nightingale image were apparent. I examined these findings in Chapter 2 and remarked that they were of particular interest to recruitment officers at national and institutional level. With a falling population of 18-year-old women from which student nurses were traditionally recruited and a declining interest in nursing as a career, the nurses in the first study were fast disappearing as a distinct group. One important question in the '90s was whether the predominant image of nursing as women's traditional work would have to change. Evidence from the recruitment literature and posters of the time suggests recruiters recognized that it did. The technical aspects of nursing were given a higher profile, and men and older women were targeted as potential recruits (Department of Health 1990).

These trends have been borne out by the demographic profile of current students both in terms of the four fieldwork sites in the subsequent study and nationally. Since 1984 the profile has clearly changed in terms of age and maturity. Awareness of gender issues, diversity and race are more explicit in government policy and educational curricula than in the 1980s, but in some ways this can drive the articulation of such issues underground by taking them for granted and normalizing them. The evaluation from a conference on the future of nursing,[1] held in spring 2010, threw up a surprising trend. Some delegates were concerned that the feminist stance adopted by some speakers in relation to nursing as a predominantly female profession, might run the risk of marginalizing the male delegates.

With regards to race and ethnicity, research undertaken in the mid-2000s on both student learning (Allan et al. 2008a) and the experiences of overseas trained nurses working in the UK health and social care systems (Smith et al. 2006) revealed that strong pockets of racial discrimination still existed. At least Mary Seacole, the Jamaican-Scottish nurse, who was working in the Crimea at the same time as Nightingale, has enjoyed increasing visibility since my first book was published. Her portraits now hang in the Royal College of Nursing and the National Portrait Gallery in London, and she was voted the 'top black Briton' of all time in 2004. Further recognition has been given to Mary Seacole by naming buildings after her and establishing centres for nursing research and practice and leadership and development awards in her name. However a national campaign to raise money for a memorial statue is slow, and to date there is no single statue in the whole of the UK dedicated to a named black woman. This state of affairs speaks for itself in terms of wider racial politics and hidden history (Green 2010).

At the beginning of the 2000s New Labour succeeded in increasing the nursing and midwifery workforce as part of their commitment to the NHS Plan. Student nurse recruitment also increased as part of that strategy but so also did student attrition, particularly among entrants in the school leaver age groups. Figures at the beginning of 2010 revealed that attrition had increased to as much as 30 per cent in some regions of the UK. Reasons for dropout were attributed to two factors: students encountering financial difficulties and faulty selection procedures.

At the time of writing the first book, the former high prestige teaching hospitals (now redefined in a clustering of hospitals as Foundation Trusts with university connections) there had always been more than enough young female applicants willing to work for low wages. Even so, despite being recruited in Nightingale's image, the City nurses of the first study resented being seen by patients as 'angels' and vocationally motivated. Most of them saw themselves as workers who were doing a job.

Students in the subsequent study were frank they had selected nursing for a variety of reasons. A number of them had previously worked as HCAs while others wanted to do more people-orientated work and saw nursing as an opportunity to acquire new skills. These students brought a depth of maturity and a wealth of life and work experience which appeared to give them the emotional capacity or competence to put themselves in other people's shoes allowing them to empathize with others including the trained staff. As one student said 'life experience gives you common sense which if you come straight from school you don't have!' Former HCAs said they wanted to study to be nurses because they felt there was 'only so far you can go' without the registered nurse qualification; gaining National Vocational Qualifications was not enough. They described how they had taken a drop in salary to become nurses and were prepared 'to go that extra mile!' As one respondent said 'you don't get a lot of thanks or money' which flew in the face of the 1990s poster about the emotional rewards of becoming a nurse or the more recent 2005 poster prioritizing the financial rewards of studying nursing at university. Students who were 18-year-old school leavers also expressed a commitment to undertaking people-orientated work. Those who opted to study for a degree rather than a diploma saw it as offering them greater career opportunities.

At what cost care?

In the first book, a 1990s recruitment poster sent a double message: that nursing offered two sorts of rewards, emotional and financial. But was the emotional component of caring adequately recognized and remunerated? I suggested in Chapter 1 that at the time of writing the first book this was not the case. I speculated that health planners and managers of the new-look health service would be so concerned with fine tuning their budgets that nurses could find themselves with increasing workloads leaving them with little time to do anything but meet patients' physical and technical needs. Emotional care was not easily costed, which put it in danger of being marginalized even further as health care moved to the market place. It could be further argued that the introduction of market-style health care reforms laid the foundation for the current focus on targets which has put pressure on the workforce to increase patient throughput.

Ironically, as I wrote in the early '90s private health insurance schemes tended to advertise their services through images of smiling nurses but without paying them any extra for the emotional component of care. I suggested that only a recruitment crisis would increase the importance of nurses' pay. By the 2000s however, the delegation of personal care to HCAs paid for at the lowest band of the Agenda for Change framework confirms that work primarily seen as care work continues to be poorly remunerated. Personal care is separated out from technical, managerial and academic expertise which in turn reinforces the hierarchy of values between different types of skills and activities illustrative of Hochschild's argument that the 'cold modern option' to learn to do without care will predominate if it is not adequately recognized, valued and adequately rewarded (Hochschild 2003).

So the image of the smiling nurse persists. In 2008 this image was very much apparent in the public sector with compassion and smiles being placed very firmly on the UK National Health Service Agenda. A press release stressed the importance of nurses' compassion and smiles to ensure patients received good care to aid their recovery while an article *'Nurses to be rated on how compassionate and smiley they are'* made front-page news in a national newspaper (Carvel 2008). Once again it appeared that nurses were being asked to smile and be compassionate over and above their 'normal' workload to meet targets and increase patient throughput without any compensatory benefits, rewards or support.

The privatization of the health service has not taken place on the scale that I predicted when the first book was published in 1992. This was partly because in 1997 a Labour government was elected committed to the publically funded NHS. Instead a mixture of quasi-privatized and market-like reforms begun during the conservative era of Thatcher and Major were continued. Some critics accused 'New Labour' of privatizing by stealth (www.lookafterournhs.org.uk). Although the health service continues to be free from 'cradle to grave' at the point of access a financial tone manifest in targets and increased patient throughput was introduced and 'experienced by the grass roots'. Students in my study were aware of the four-hour targets to get patients through the emergency department to either discharge or admission, and they reported that sometimes it felt like beds rather than patients were being managed.

With the announcement of savage budget cuts by the coalition government in November 2010 and radical reform in the public sector there are fears that UK health and social care is about to enter a period of extreme austerity and privatization predicted in the White Paper *Equity and Excellence: Liberating the NHS* (Department of Health 2010a), adding further weight to Hochschild's 'cold modern' option of learning to live without care.

The future of nursing theory and practice

When the clinical career structure was introduced in 1988 a new future for nurses was envisaged with the potential to reward clinical skills and responsibilities. Over half-a-million nursing jobs were re-graded over a period of six months. But many nurses were disappointed with their grading and often found themselves competing with colleagues for a limited number of posts because of inadequate funding. Despite the difficulties, however, the re-grading process showed the potential for rewarding nurses for their expertise and improving their career structure (Beardshaw and Robinson 1990).

The planned reforms for nurse education set out by the United Kingdom Central Council's (UKCC) Project 2000 (UKCC 1986) were closely associated with the changes taking place in nursing's clinical career structure. As a consequence of the educational reforms, the three-year hospital-based programme, during which students spent the majority of their time on the wards as the principal workforce and only 30 weeks in the classroom, was described in the first study as giving way to American-style college programmes and supernumerary clinical status.

The follow-up study was able to provide insights into the implications of supernumerary status for students who had undertaken Project 2000 programmes and more recently the Fitness for Practice curriculum. Students described how they negotiated their supernumerary status from placement to placement which they could not take as a given. When the ward was busy they had to be counted as part of the workforce. The study also revealed that students did not necessarily have consistent clinical teaching and had to rely on a variety of mentors as they progressed from one placement to the next, often with low input from their university link lecturers.

Developments such as Agenda for Change and Modernising Nursing Careers (Department of Health 2004a, RCN 2005, Department of Health 2006) will affect the future shape of nurses' careers and also form an integral part of the Nursing and Midwifery Council's (NMC) proposed educational programme of reforms.

Agenda for Change

Agenda for Change, introduced in 2005, evaluated jobs against sixteen factors.[2] On scrutinizing the criteria for elements of emotional labour, only two were explicitly related to emotional aspects of care. These were: 1. 'Communication and relationship skills' and 15. 'Emotional effort' i.e. 'Are there any emotional demands associated with your role?' The others were associated with knowledge, skills and responsibilities. The rationale for the scheme was to ensure that nurses were fairly evaluated in relation to their expertise and paid accordingly across nine bands from HCA to nurse consultant. The job evaluation had to be further assessed against the NHS Knowledge and Skills Framework (KSF) which formed an integral part of the pre-registration educational curriculum.

The Agenda for Change reinforces the discourse of nursing and caring which manifests itself as the sharp division of labour between HCAs who give personal care, students who are learning to be registered nurses and registered nurses who undertake drug rounds, dressings and other technical and management activities. Student nurses equate 'caring' to personal patient care which is HCAs' work rather than nursing work. Nursing is synonymous with technical tasks and valuable to students' learning because they see it as integral to their future role whereas HCA work equates to being used 'as a pair of hands'.

However HCAs are vital to the health care workforce. They are also in a unique position to give insights into contemporary nursing as the people who work closest to the registered nurse. In one study trained nurses told HCAs how they feared losing their connections with patients as their role became more technical while ward managers risked becoming 'more like accountants' (Knibb et al. 2006). In the same study an enlightened ward manager conceptualized the work of registered nurses and HCAs working alongside each other, in a holistic way, each contributing their respective skills 'as a group of people who work together as one workforce'. This insight points the way ahead for the future of nursing care and nurses' capacity to care as a holistic workforce.

Modernising nursing careers

The need to review the future direction of pre- and post-registration nurse education alongside the modernizing nursing careers initiative reflected the NMC's recognition of the changes in the UK health environment where people are living longer with multiple long-term conditions and continuing health inequalities. The NMC worked with government departments in the four UK countries to develop a framework for nursing based on patient groups, rather than specific medical conditions, and the settings where they are cared for. The proposed career framework is mapped against family and public health, mental health and psychosocial care, supporting long-term care and acute and critical care, from staff nurse (Band 5) through to directors and professors (Band 9). This framework marks a departure from the career structure of the '80s, which was organized around clinical specialities.

The framework is represented diagrammatically by two tools, which are designed to encompass areas of care rather than individual diseases and conditions. The tools are currently being developed to be used on-line with the aim to (1) assist nurses to 'care for your future in nursing' and (2) provide service managers with a framework to 'shape a quality nursing workforce'. Both nurses and managers are advised to always emphasize 'promoting health and illness prevention' among 'children, young people, adults and older people'. It is interesting to see nursing language returning to an emphasis on health and illness prevention despite what many would regard as the failure of Project 2000 to establish a philosophy of health as a basis for pre-registration nurse education and practice (Smith et al. 1995).

As this book goes to press in 2011 the modernization programme to facilitate workforce transformation is nearing completion with the added impetus to 'drive forward the ambitions' of the coalition government's *Equity and Excellence* White Paper (Modernising Nursing Careers, 2011, http://www.dh.gov.uk/en/Aboutus/Chiefprofessionalofficers/Chiefnursingofficer/DH_108368, Department of Health 2010a).

Maintaining morale and wellbeing

In the 1980s, a survey of British nursing investigated factors affecting recruitment and retention (Price Waterhouse 1988). Respondents were particularly dissatisfied with low staffing levels, heavy workloads and inadequate standards of care. Two decades later similar trends were identified in the ward learning environment questionnaire. Both qualitative and quantitative responses suggested that student nurses found those learning environments particularly challenging when staffing levels were inadequate for the workload, which limited their learning and the quality of care they felt able to give. On the contrary, a positive association was found between the item 'The workload does not interfere with teaching or learning' and placement satisfaction indicated by student perceptions of 'happiness' and 'learning opportunities'. These findings were taken as indicators that students' 'supernumerary' status had been recognized. They were also positively associated with students' perceptions of quality of patient care.

The connection between student, staff and patient morale was clearly demonstrated by Revans (1964) and was the inspiration for my original study of student learning and caring. Indeed I concluded then and since that 'What is good for nurses is good for patients' (Lowes 2010). A similar connection was made in a major review of staff health and wellbeing which showed that when the health service was well managed 'staff felt more valued and respected', and sickness and absence rates were reduced (Batty 2010). In particular the Accident and Emergency department of one trust and 'arguably the most stressful' was singled out for its low staff sickness and high retention which was attributed to it being 'well managed'. The review concluded that maintaining a healthy engaged workforce was necessary to ensure the delivery of high quality care but that this relationship was likely to be undermined by financial cutbacks that put staff under increasing pressure to do more for less.

Emotions, experiential learning and new knowledge

The application of my original findings in the 1980s and '90s was of particular relevance to the content and form of the then new style pre-registration training with its emphasis on people and health rather than patients and disease. Findings presented in chapters 3 and 4 of the first book offer important perspectives on the knowledge base of nursing as 'people work' and its relationship between ward and classroom. They show, for example, how nurses defined the physical, technical and emotional components of their clinical work according to medical specialities and attached importance to 'liking' some patients more than others. The findings also show that students frequently found themselves in emotionally charged situations which went beyond the medical and technical definitions of their training and back to nursing as 'people work' in which they engaged in emotional labour. Often they experienced anxiety and stress because their emotional labour went largely unrecognized and undervalued as part of 'real' nursing. Neither was it incorporated into the theoretical and practical organization of their training.

On the basis of these findings I suggested that the emotional components of caring require formal and systematic training to manage feelings, grounded in a theoretical base such as psychology, sociology and the acquisition of complex interpersonal skills. In this way emotion work would be made visible and valued in its own right and not viewed as *just* part of the package of women's work. To some extent this has happened in terms of rhetoric and documentation as described in the earlier chapters of this book although gender still remains a contested and marginalized issue.

In the 1980s, nurse academics were also proposing nursing theories that went beyond the conceptual limitations of the nursing process. I noted at the time that these developments held possibilities for using research findings from studies such as mine to build an empirically tested knowledge base rooted in practice. It is interesting that Alan Pearson, founder of the first UK Nursing Development Unit (Pearson 1988) and professor of evidence-based health care, when asked to name a piece of 'life-changing research' to mark the fiftieth anniversary of the Royal College of Nursing's research society, identified the emotional labour research undertaken by Nicky James and myself (Pearson 2009, p. 19). He said:

> In examining the core nature of nursing they (Smith and James) reveal that, although engagement in the practicalities of physical caring and curing is a critical component of nursing, the 'labour' of nurses is intrinsically emotional and requires the nurse to participate emotionally with those she or he cares for .

Pearson concluded that although emotional labour was:

> Just one of many new understandings to have emerged from the past 50 years of research, it has influenced me greatly as I grapple with the subtleties and complexities of excellent nursing practice.

As I discuss in Chapter 1, the research on emotions and the use of emotional labour as a device for understanding care has been developed and consolidated since the 1980s. More specifically Freshwater and Stickley's (2004) position paper critiques the current state of the nurse education curriculum and supports the case for teaching emotional intelligence to counter the limitations inherent in the requirements of a curriculum subject to NMC regulations and reflected in a classroom dominated by propositional 'textbook' knowledge as distinct from the practical knowledge acquired in clinical settings (2004, p. 92).

Emotional intelligence in Freshwater and Stickley's view allows for balancing the rational with the emotional and for emphasizing the emotional components of caring: the empathy, the relationships and interpersonal communication reflected in a curriculum that encompassed the complexity of human interaction and patient-centred care. They make the connection with some of the early nursing theorists: Peplau (1992), Newman (1994) and Parse (1997) – who provided theoretical substance to this complexity. While agreeing that nursing needs an emotionally intelligent curriculum Freshwater and Stickley do not mention the emotional labour literature nor take on board some of the latest critiques of emotional intelligence as a tool of management that resides in the realms of cognitive rather than emotional understanding. Rather they hark back to Menzies' classic work as the touch point for all subsequent emotional understanding. In summary the emotions literature has been opened out by a series of key studies that over the years has built on the profundity and impact of Menzies' original research (1960). Freshwater and Stickley's position reflects the critiques and perceived limitations of emotional labour as a conceptual device for understanding the deeper aspects of emotional work, most notably relational caring and empathy and the giving of emotional care, as a 'gift' rather than a conscious commodity. Theodosius (2008) has further extended the analysis of emotional labour by applying psychoanalytic theory to examine the nature of emotions that nurses feel and how they form a part of their social identity which goes beyond the presentational symbolic forms expressed through the emotion management framework first inspired by Hochschild (1983).

On the topic of nursing research more generally over the past two decades there has been a greater recognition and integration of research as part of nursing encouraged by the move to higher education on the one hand and participation in research that is internationally recognized on the other (Lipsett 2008).[3]

Could this be regarded as the legacy of the UKCC's Project 2000 which took nursing into the higher education sector and was committed to preparing practitioners who were 'knowledgeable doers' and teaching students 'how to learn and how to analyse, to give them confidence and the motivation and facilities to develop themselves in relation to a changing environment' (UKCC, 1985, p. 21)? The UKCC's recommendations certainly encouraged nurses to re-examine traditional definitions of nursing knowledge, teaching and learning based on notions of tacit knowledge which is uncodified and transmitted through tone, feel and expression (Collins, 1974, Eraut, 1985, p. 119).

Benner's (1984) classic text suggests ways in which tacit knowledge is developed, by describing how nurses move through five stages from 'novice' to 'expert'. The use of intuition in decision making distinguishes the 'expert' nurse practitioner from the beginner. The endurance of Benner's framework and popularity among the nursing community was still evident in the Chief Nurse for England, Chris Beasley's introduction to the Department of Health's consultation on Modernising Nursing Careers in which she suggested to nurses that in their post-registration careers they should '"major" in one pathway moving from "novice to expert"' (Department of Health 2007).

In later writings, Benner and others describe how intuition is developed through and used in clinical practice:

> It is the unique, remarkable capacity of the body to cope with vague, 'fuzzy' information and regions of influence and tension that makes possible the human capacity to function in ambiguous, underdetermined situations (Benner and Wrubel 1989, p. 53).

Indeed the importance of integrating intuitive insights with systematic knowledge has been increasingly recognized since the 1980s (Sheehan 1983). Eraut has continued to develop his thinking on tacit knowledge and in recent research he has captured knowledge from the academic, organizational and practice context. More specifically, he has looked at the needs of newly qualified nurses, accountants and engineers (Eraut et al. 2007). Furthermore approaches such as Eraut's are especially appropriate to recognizing emotional labour as a key component of nursing, requiring the acquisition of a set of hitherto uncodified skills. Evans and colleagues built on Eraut's research to develop the notion of 'putting knowledge to work' for practice-based disciplines to show how students can apply and interrogate formal knowledge learnt in the classroom and integrate it in practice (Evans et al. 2009, Evans et al. 2010).

The findings presented in chapter 5 of the first book were of key importance in understanding emotional labour as part of the labour process of nursing and the conditions necessary for its production and reproduction in the workplace. When nurses felt appreciated and supported emotionally by their ward sisters, they not only had role models for emotionally explicit patient care but they also felt better able to care for patients in this way. Patients and nurses were sensitive to ward atmospheres and social relations created by the sisters. The assumption was that technical and physical labour would be enhanced when underpinned by an emotionally explicit caring style. The nursing process philosophy and work method created greater emotional involvement for students than task allocation. It also potentially increased their anxiety. This finding was of particular relevance, given the move across the UK as part of the 'New

Nursing' to introduce primary nursing as a cornerstone initiative of Nursing Development Units which went beyond the recommendations of the nursing process in promoting continuity of care (Pearson 1988, Salvage 1990, Jones and Bamford 1998). Primary nursing further raised the profile of emotional care by placing even greater emphasis on interpersonal relationships between nurses and individual patients. Some primary nurses identified the need for supervision as used by psychiatric nurses and social workers if primary nursing were to be effective (Johns 1990). So it is interesting that two decades later Alan Pearson, founder of the first Nursing Development Unit, identified the importance of emotional labour research as being particularly significant in understanding nursing's subtleties and complexities (Pearson op. cit.). But why does primary nursing no longer feature in the 2000s? Benton's view is that UK market reforms made it too costly as a way of organizing nursing care (Benton 2004).

The disappearing ward sister

In the 1980s, wards where ward sisters had an express commitment to a person-centred approach to care, articulated through the use of the nursing process or primary nursing as a work method, were more likely to create the infrastructure which allowed the production and reproduction of emotional labour. The sister's personal work preferences and priorities were more important in shaping the content of the nurses' work and learning than the medical labels of the wards (cf. Fretwell 1982). The sister's emotional style of management was the key to the well-being of patients and nurses.

As mentioned at the beginning of this book one of the motivations to undertake a follow-up study was to find out who was currently leading the clinical learning during students' practice placements. The study revealed that the ward sister's role had become fragmented and was being undertaken by a variety of clinical nurses under the ward manager's leadership who at his/her most effective was continuing to undertake emotional labour 'at a distance' to create a positive learning and caring environment.

In 2009 a Royal College of Nursing (RCN) investigation of the role of the ward sister/charge nurse found that their increased leadership responsibilities prevented them from directly supervising clinical practice so that they were unable to directly oversee standards of care within the ward environment (RCN 2009). The RCN concluded that in the context of the NHS quality agenda, this was not acceptable and that work needed to be undertaken to strengthen and support the role. A prime ministerial commission on frontline care reinforced this view and further recommended that the traditional role of the ward sister should be restored with immediate steps being taken 'to strengthen this role and enhance its clinical leadership and visible authority as the guardian of patient safety and the role model for the next generation of nursing students' (Prime Minister's Commission 2010).

In Chapter 5 I describe how the mentor rather than the traditional ward sister has become the students' role model. In some instances ward managers or sisters also acted as mentors but this was by no means the case. One practice educator (PE) observed that although how a ward was run overall had a bearing on a student's learning, 'When you talk to students if they've had a very good mentor that seems to swing it for them; their mentor is the greatest influence of all'.

Death and dying in hospital: still the ultimate emotional labour

Many of the issues explored in previous chapters were drawn together in Chapter 6 in order to further the understanding of emotional labour as a concept and its organization in the hospital ward. Here I was particularly interested in how nurses in hospitals managed the ultimate emotional labour in caring for people who were dying, given that hospital was still the most likely place where people died. But as Field (1989) points out, busy hospital wards are not necessarily the most suitable place to die, and many people would prefer to stay at home but for the inadequacy of the community services. In the 1980s I found, as with other situations in which emotional labour was called for, that the ward sister's role was fundamental in putting death, dying and bereavement on the ward agenda. I also found that because students' feelings were rarely acknowledged in the open arena of the ward nor adequately addressed within their formal training, they developed distancing strategies to keep them from involvement. They were unwilling to accept that they could be formally taught to 'react', preferring to see their learning about death and dying as experiential.

As I noted in the new version of Chapter 6 there has been a greater recognition of death and dying in the media, and a succession of research studies have provided the material to inform both curricula and practice. As the dying process becomes protracted among the increasing numbers of people suffering with long-term conditions, the National Institute of Clinical Excellence (NICE) guidelines and the Cancer Charities recognize that palliative care needs to be integrated across the whole spectrum of care, not just at the end of life. Hospital continues to be the place where most people die although initiatives such as the Liverpool Care Pathway (LCP) have been introduced 'to provide an evidence based framework for the delivery of appropriate care for dying patients and their relatives in a variety of settings'. Ironically the framework may also provide a mechanism for helping students to emotionally distance themselves from the dying process.

Facilitating caring trajectories

In Chapter 3 I described each pre-registration curriculum in place at the time of the two studies. In the 2000s, the UK population's changing and increasingly complex health needs are important factors driving the need to review nurse education. The current curriculum is now undergoing a major review in preparation for degree-only programmes by September 2013. Future pre-registration programmes will have two progression points, the first of which students will be expected to meet basic care and safety criteria at the same time as demonstrating 'professional behaviours'. The second progression point requires students to show that they can work more independently, confidently and safely while demonstrating critical thinking skills (NMC 2010a). The new programmes will combine a mix of generic and 'field' specific skills to cover the spheres of practice envisioned by the modernized nursing career framework.

Chapter 7 describes the students' caring trajectories and originally looked at the factors that shaped their emotional careers. Students described trajectories where they begin fresh and enthusiastic with an 'uncanny way' of getting to know their patients, but arrived at the end of three years' training 'cynical and disillusioned'. A number of caring factors were identified which influenced students' caring styles and capacity over time and their choice of future forms of emotional labour. Personal support was *ad hoc* throughout training, and personal relationships were fragmented between nurses and nurses and patients aggravated by the shift and allocation systems. I speculated that if students' individuality and caring commitment is repressed too often and for too long then it is likely that they will choose hierarchical relations, stereotyping and labelling as preferred forms of emotional labour.

Melia (1984, 1987) noted the discontinuity suffered by student nurses. Their rapid movement from ward to ward and shift to shift, as I found, militated against them working with the same nurse (trained or untrained) for any length of time. Much attention was given to this problem by the Project 2000 working groups, and it was expected that students who are now supernumerary would be allocated to fewer clinical areas and for longer periods where they required close supervision and support. The English National Board (1987), for example, suggested that 'each student must have a named supervisor or mentor in each practical placement'. On the basis of the findings of my first study I supported this recommendation for students to have a clearly identified person responsible for their teaching and assessment in each clinical allocation. However, I made a number of comments at that time. One issue I identified was whether the person was called a supervisor or a mentor since I found that students felt uncomfortable with the idea of being 'supervised' in the sense of being 'checked every inch of the way'. Given the importance of the nursing hierarchy in shaping relationships, and their fragmentary and discontinuous nature, three important recommendations emerged from my first study. One was that student nurses should be able to choose their supervisor/mentor; secondly this person should not be hierarchically threatening to them; and thirdly they should be able to continue their relationship throughout the students' training.

I then suggested that the duties of the mentor go far beyond those of the supervisor as teacher and assessor. The mentor needed to encourage and help shape the career of her student and be caring and able to offer advice and direction in the face of problems. She must also be an acknowledged expert in her own right (Bracken and Davies 1989). Thus the mentor would make intelligible the students' learning experiences and provide them with support systems that both enabled them to recognize and undertake emotional labour in a positive way. As the subsequent research and other studies have since shown, these qualities still hold fast today.

At the time of the first study, the most likely people to supervise the students were either senior student nurses or recently qualified staff nurses. The staff nurses were prepared for their role by post-basic teaching and assessing courses validated by the national training boards. There were not enough of them either to take on these roles or with the necessary personal and professional experience to do them well.

The UKCC was aware that measures needed to be taken to help trained nurses to meet the challenges generated by changes in education and practice such as proposals developed by the Post-Registration Education and Practice Project (PREPP) (UKCC 1990). The project recommended ways of keeping practitioners up to date and preparing newly registered nurses to take on their new responsibilities. Newly qualified nurses were recommended to have a period of support from designated 'preceptors' who were sufficiently experienced to 'act as a role model' and 'evolve individual and learning methods in a flexible relationship'. In 2010, the introduction of preceptors for newly registered nurses was again recommended, this time as part of the modernization agenda (Department of Health 2010b).

The student nurse mentorship system first proposed by the UKCC and subsequently formalized by its successor, the NMC, stipulates that the student's placement outcomes must only be signed off by a qualified 'sign off' mentor who may work in conjunction with an associate mentor (NMC 2008b, NMC 2010c). The NMC also stipulates an educational route for clinical nurses to participate in formal mentor training and a pathway that leads to qualification as a nurse lecturer. Since students have become supernumerary, their relationship with their mentor has become particularly crucial. In Chapter 5 I identified the qualities that students valued in their mentors and the conditions necessary to establish a good relationship with them. I also showed that other conditions essential to successful mentorship, recommended in my first book, had not come to fruition. The result is that students do not choose their mentors; the role of mentor and assessor is not distinct; there is no continuity between student and mentor from one placement to the next. On the contrary students relate to a succession of mentors during their three-year programme. It became clear however that a positive mentoring relationship was the key to student learning and created a 'humanistic approach' to each placement.

In order to ensure that registered nurses become effective student mentors and preceptors to newly qualified staff, the importance of early career training is evident in Eraut and colleagues' (2007) study of early career learning in nursing, engineering and accounting. The researchers found that in all three professions the new graduates' work profiles and experiences were extremely complex and varied, resulting in them being either under or overly challenged. The complexity and variety of their work appeared to be related to their individual recognition of and input to their learning but also the different learning opportunities they encountered. Nurses as a group were found to be the least supported on qualifying, and they were consistently over challenged physically, mentally and emotionally as they faced increased responsibility and work pressures in most clinical environments. Support and feedback were critically important for all groups to assist learning, improve retention and maintain their commitment. Nurses in particular found difficulty in negotiating the time to attend Continuing Professional Development (CPD) or coaching sessions (similar to being allocated a preceptor), made even more difficult by the lack of potential coaches. The ward manager was identified as the individual who could either enhance or hinder this situation. The importance of regular feedback and mutual support was identified for all groups. To be effective, feedback had to take place in the context of good workplace relationships in order to encourage strengths and work on weaknesses to meet organizational expectations. The research also recommended that 'the emotional dimension of working life requires ongoing attention' (Eraut et al. 2007).

These findings are particularly relevant for pre-registration and undergraduate students and confirm the importance of emotions and relationships in workplace learning. They also support nursing policies and practices which espouse the importance of skilled mentors and preceptors to facilitate the caring trajectories of students and newly qualified staff in order to produce and reproduce the emotional labour of nursing from one generation of nurses to the next.

The effects of emotional care on patient outcomes

In the conclusion to my first book, I gave the final words to the patients. One reason was to address the question that I imagined was on the lips of general managers looking for cost-effectiveness and efficiency. What effect did emotional labour have on patient outcomes? Positive forms of emotional labour certainly made them feel better. And there was sufficient evidence that negative forms of emotional labour which stereotyped and labelled patients could be positively harmful. A case in point was a television docu-drama which caused a great stir among the public and hospital world alike when it was broadcast in the early 00s. It was called 'Major Implications' (MacMillan 1980). It was about a woman who was admitted to hospital for minor surgery and ended up having a large proportion of her bowel removed. What happened was the following. The woman, a successful middle-class artist, divorced with two children with a new partner, decided to have a sterilization. It became clear from the beginning that the nurses did not approve of her decision. They were coldly polite to her. On return from surgery she did not recover as quickly as was expected. On the first postoperative day she was encouraged, according to the routine, to get up and wash herself. The nurses dismissed her complaints of nausea and were not even sympathetic when she fainted. Because they did not approve of her and resented her middle-class articulateness they labelled her as a 'difficult patient'. Consequently they failed to take her complaints seriously. The doctors reacted similarly, and there was collusion between them and the nurses. Eventually, after five days of decline, culminating in the frank symptoms of intestinal obstruction, the unfortunate woman was rushed to the operating theatre. Part of her bowel had to be excised, and she was left with a permanent colostomy and a ruined life. If the nurses had looked beyond the stereotype they might have saved her physical and emotional suffering.

But when nurses engaged in positive emotional labour their effects on their patients were profound, as the following account, by a cancer patient, demonstrates.

P.   When I discovered my diagnosis, I wanted to share it or get rid of it if you like. If I try to hide things then that just makes matters worse.

Q.   Do you feel you've had permission to do that ... ?

P.   Yes. The nurses have been brilliant. They're such good listeners. They've held my hand literally and metaphorically. They've said exactly the right things at the right time. I've never been patronized by either the doctors or nurses. If I felt they were hiding something that would make me worry and effect me emotionally and probably physically as well. After I'd been here a few days the nurses must have guessed that I needed to talk. They'd obviously read my notes. One nurse came to me and we held hands, it was a real comfort. It's difficult to describe but there was no fear. It was so natural and it had a calming influence even though I cried. It happened on two different occasions. But to give yourself a chance physically you need to have the emotional side there helping you.

The patient made clear links between the emotional and physical aspects of her care. She described caring gestures, the little things that make her feel qualitatively different: nurses who recognized she needed to talk, were good listeners, held her hand, took away her fear and had a calming influence on her. She described them as 'brilliant', indicating that she recognized they had skills, but also implied that these caring gestures were 'natural', both in the sense of intuitive and genuine. Emotional labour made a difference and care mattered to patients, back then and still does but remains in danger of being marginalized.

The skill lies in the nurse who is able to recognize that emotional labour is needed and may be required in different forms for different patients. Not everyone wants to hold hands and show their tears in front of others. Would the emotional labour have taken a different form if the genders of the actors were reversed or their class, race and cultures were different? Did the patient make a better recovery from surgery than if she hadn't been emotionally supported in this way? Had the nurses been formally taught to listen and recognize the patient's need to talk? How did they feel after their encounter, and who supported them and gave them feedback?

In response to my own analysis I wrote that there was clearly scope for much more research in the area of emotion and health care. The pressure was and is clearly on to intensify nursing work in a new wave of changes in nurses' education, work organization and NHS managers looking to their budgets. Nurses are at the frontline of care, and they do make a difference as my first book showed.

In this second book I have interrogated the original findings and updated them with new research designed to follow up and specifically to find out what has happened to the ward sister role and who leads caring and learning in the clinical setting in a dramatically changed policy, political, organizational and educational context.

I conclude with two inquiries into the care provided by the Maidstone and Tunbridge Wells NHS Trust (Health Care Commission 2007) and the Mid Staffordshire NHS Foundation Trust (Francis 2010a). To some extent the results of the inquiries could be seen as representing the flip side of emotional labour, the compassionate care index, emotional touch points and the consequences of policy drivers in which nurses and nursing care become the lens and potential scapegoats through which difficult issues are revealed. These two inquiries have become defining moments in the history of the new NHS with its financial tone manifest in targets and rapid patient throughput. The inquiries certainly revealed that pressure on management to meet targets and financial imperatives had impacted on the quality of care. The physical environments of both organizations were seen as problematic, and in the case of Maidstone and Tunbridge Wells the spread of the Clostridium Difficile infection was partly attributed to the lack of facilities to isolate infected patients effectively. Quality of nursing care came under scrutiny in both organizations, where for a variety of reasons nurses appeared to be unable to provide nursing care that both responded to patients' physical and emotional needs. Furthermore staff, relatives and patients lived in an atmosphere of fear to speak out about the failures in care in case there were reprisals for their ongoing care. Student nurses and their tutors were also asked whether they noticed anything amiss during their placements and whether they had a responsibility to speak out (Brindle 2010). The Chair of the Mid-Staffordshire inquiry stated:

> The Inquiry found that a chronic shortage of staff, particularly nursing staff, was largely responsible for the substandard care. Morale at the Trust was low, and while many staff did their best in difficult circumstances, others showed a disturbing lack of compassion towards their patients. Staff who spoke out felt ignored and there is strong evidence that many were deterred from doing so through fear and bullying. (Francis 2010b)

There are resonances in this statement with the emotional labour analysis where in order for patients to feel safe and cared for the staff who care for them must also feel safe and cared for. The difference in the nursing and health-care world of the twenty-first century from when I first reported my emotional labour study is that the effects of emotions on individuals, groups and organizations are more likely to be recognized and talked about. Nurses need to be equipped with critical, emotional and intellectual skills in order to work in a complex, global world and lead care in hospital or home, residential home or hospice.

I will leave the final word to Sister Ronda who was the original inspiration for the emotional labour analysis of my first study. Her father had died recently, following a long period of failing health. Reflecting on his last 24 hours in hospital Sister Ronda described how he received 'the most wonderful loving care, which made me very proud of the nursing profession'. When I asked what was it that made her 'very proud' she said it was the way in which the staff responded to her father's rapidly changing condition, making themselves available during such a difficult, unpredictable and emotional time. Although the ward was a short stay medical assessment unit with fast patient throughput she found this did not detract from a ward ethos that was 'so helpful from the top down'. Sister Ronda described one particular staff nurse whose knowledge of pain control and recognition of 'the little things' ensured Mr Ronda's comfort, as well as supporting her to be with him as he lay dying and when he died. It later turned out that this staff nurse had been through such a traumatic experience when her own parent died, and she was determined to ensure patients and families should only receive the very best end-of-life care possible. And she was able to do this because the senior sister was always there in the background promoting an ethos of care.

By revisiting the original data and the notion of emotional labour presented in the first book I have been able to scrutinize new evidence to show that nurses can still care but that it requires effort, skill and organizational support. Sister Ronda's account certainly confirms this view. But care has become a contested concept because of policy and organizational changes that have hierarchically spilt nursing between qualified nurses and HCAs. Nurses and nursing therefore need more than ever the support and commitment of leaders who set an emotionally caring tone and promote an organizational and educational system sensitive to the complex and financially driven world of the twenty-first century.

Notes

Preface

1. Ward sister' and 'sister' are equivalent to 'charge nurse'.

Foreword

1 In nursing homes too, privatization has brought bad news. A recent review in the *British Medical Journal* reviewed 40 studies comparing private with non-private nursing homes, and concluded that for-profit nursing homes suffered high staff turnover, fewer hours of care, and are actually more likely to die early than patients – in the same medical condition – living in not-for-profit nursing homes. Vikram R. Comondore et al., 'Quality of care in for-profit and not-for-profit nursing homes: Systematic review and meta-analysis' *British Medical Journal* 339 (2009). See Hochschild, *The Outsourced Self: Intimate Life in Market Times*, New York: Metropolitan Press, forthcoming.

I Introduction

1. How do student nurses learn to care? A review of the literature and a case study into whether changes in nurse education and health care organisation have influenced the ways in which student nurses learn in the new NHS. Short title: Leadership for Learning. Funded by the General Nursing Council Trust for England and Wales and the Centre for Research in Nursing and Midwifery Education, The University of Surrey, undertaken by Helen Allan, Pam Smith, Mike O'Driscoll and Maria Lorentzon. Ethical clearance to undertake the research was obtained before data collection commenced. The study began in January 2006 and was completed in December 2007.
2. Educational role introduced to support the student's clinical learning either directly or indirectly in conjunction with the mentor. Magnusson and colleagues (2007) observe that role descriptions and titles differ, but they have the common aim of improving and strengthening student nurses' practice learning.
3. The Nursing and Midwifery Council specifies that the mentor's role is to be accountable for decisions to delegate work to students while maintaining their supernumerary status as part of the Council's remit to protect the public.
4. Evidence of 'lack of care' in long-stay institutions includes a study of work organisation and social relations in a geriatric hospital (Evers 1981a, 1984). The findings of a number of studies quoted by Evers summarize life in a geriatric hospital as routinized physical care; harassed nurses battling against the clock; depersonalization of patients to the status of work objects. Evers uses the notion of 'warehousing', i.e. care at its most routine and depersonalized as distinct from a 'horticultural' model which encourages individuality, which was first conceptualized by Miller and Gwynne (1972) in a study of institutional care for the disabled.

5. The 'little things' are the victims of what Davies (1990) and other writers call competing rationalities which underpin institutionalized care work. Scientific and technical-economic rationalities correspond to male-orientated doctor and administrator 'assembly line care of the sick'. Costs are kept to a minimum, and as many patients as possible are processed through medical diagnosis and treatment in the minimum time possible. Female caring activities are motivated by a responsibility or nurturing rationality where 'response to human need', often through the so-called little things, is paramount. In institutionalized care, however, where scientific and technical-economic rationalities dominate, these 'little things' are neither recognized nor costed into the work process except by the carers who struggle to 'fit them in'. The moral and ethical dimensions of caring and the controversial question as to whether women develop a gender-specific morality are considered by Gilligan (1982) and Tronto (1987).

6. Abel-Smith (1960) suggests that nursing in the voluntary hospitals provided a suitable occupation for the daughters of the higher social classes. It was only able to do this however by promoting nursing as a 'vocation' requiring duty, devotion and obedience, the epitome of the 'good' woman. In keeping with the social relationships of Victorian middle-class society, nurses (women) were expected to be subordinate to doctors (men).

   Carpenter (1978) suggests that 'what emerged in the voluntary hospital was the reproduction of the wider Victorian class structure based on preconceived notions of the division of labour between the sexes and between women of different classes.' The ward sister or matron complemented the authority of the doctor (a man) in organizing the nurses and domestic staff in a mirror image of how, as the 'lady of the house', she would have supported her husband and supervised the servants.

7. In 2011 'Casualty' is one of the most popular and long-running UK TV series.

8. The NHS Plan (2000) supported the increase in the number of health care assistants (HCAs) and confirmed their role in the delivery of front line care. The workforce changes in the NHS were reflected in the voluntary, independent and social sectors.

9. Ungerson (1983a) draws attention to women's unpaid and unrecognized contribution to the maintenance of the British Welfare Sate. Ungerson describes how women may be involved throughout their lives in caring for others: a child, a husband, a sick, handicapped or elderly relative in a 'cycle of care'.

10. Ungerson (1983b), in line with others, claims that women have a set of skills unique to their gender. Mothering as an example of 'private' care work has much in common with institutionalized, i.e. 'public' care work.

    Davies and Rosser (1986), in a study of women working as Higher Clerical officers in the health sector, introduce the term 'gendered job' to describe how gender is built into the labour process. The job 'capitalises on the qualities and capabilities a women has gained by virtue of having lived her life as a woman'. But, like nurses, these qualities and capabilities were regarded as part of the package rather than as an essential part of the job requiring higher status and financial rewards.

11. The traditional solution reverses the changes that have taken place in women's entry into the workforce and places them very firmly back in the home with caring responsibilities. The post-modern solution demands the removal of the central image of the caring mother leaving men and women in the workforce and the need for all sectors of society to learn to live without care. The cold modern model institutionalizes all forms of human care while the warm modern model values care at the individual, family and public level typified by high levels of state investment such as in Norway and Finland.

12. Bolton (2000) identifies four types of emotion management which can be interpreted as motivational factors as in presentational (emotion management according to general social 'rules'), philanthropic (as in emotion management given as a gift), prescriptive (emotion management as prescribed by organizations/professional rules of conduct) and pecuniary (the performance of emotion management for gain).

13. Theodosius suggests ways that nurses can be supported to learn to incorporate and manage complex, messy emotions as part of who they are in terms of both their personal and professional self and draws on Archer's work on personal and social identity mediated through reflexive 'inner dialogue' to develop these theoretical perspectives (Archer 2000, cited by Theodosius, 2008: 91).

14. The nursing process has two components: the underlying philosophy that promotes a people-orientated approach to patients based on models of care such as Henderson's (1960), and Roper's (1976) living activities and a problem-solving work method. The nursing process as work method recommends the organization of nursing into four stages defined as assessment, planning, implementation and evaluation of patient care (de la Cuesta 1983).

    McFarlane (1977) in her keynote address clearly spelt out the skills that nurses would require to practise the 'process' effectively. The observational and interviewing skills spelt out by McFarlane were clearly 'people' skills, the acquisition of which was necessary if the nursing process was to become part of the nurse's 'approach and repertoire'. In the same year (1977), the nursing process appeared for the first time in the syllabus of the national nurse training curriculum (General Nursing Council, 1977). Armstrong (1983) noted that once the nursing process had become officialised in this way, the textbook presentation of the nurse's role changes. Patients were no longer described in strictly biological terms. Psychology and communication skills were emphasized, and 'subjectivity' and emotions were encouraged as part of the nurse-patient relationship.

15. Salvage (1990) dates 'new nursing' from the 1970s. A number of influences have contributed to its development: the growth of academic nursing and interest in nursing theories, the women's movement to male and US influence in redefining nurses' unique contribution to healing. An important element of new nursing is about 'transforming relationships with patients'.

16. Freidson (1970) suggests that nurses can never be completely professionally autonomous, because traditionally their knowledge and skills revolve around the diagnostic and treatment model of care. As discussed in note 6 above, doctors also control the admission of patients and their treatment. In the public's eyes nurses are often seen as doctors' assistants. They also rely on being part of the medical division of labour for their claims to being professional.

17. Salvage describes *The Politics of Nursing* as the product of years of informal and formal discussions with nurses and participation in groups such as the Radical Nurses in the early 1980s. I was a member of the group at the time, and we wanted desperately to offer an alternative analysis to mainstream views of nurses and nurses as meek, submissive and mindless.

18. Mary O'Brien (1989) defines 'male-stream' thought as 'the massive dense intellectual current of male intellectual history' as opposed to the relatively short public history of feminist understanding (p. 3) which allows women to reproduce the world in their own terms. Male-stream thought and the belief that knowledge is 'objective' and 'abstract' promotes dualism and the setting up of opposites in a systematic way. Hence mind is described as abstract, body as material, science as abstract, common sense as material, intellectual work as abstract, manual and domestic labour as material, male as abstract, female as material and so on (p. 7).

19. Kathy Curtis, doctoral student and senior tutor at the University of Surrey, is completing a study of the professional socialization of student nurses, and the factors impacting upon development of knowledge and skills related to compassionate nursing under my and Dr Khim Horton's supervision. A doctoral studentship in Compassion in Care research has been established at the University of Huddersfield in 2011 in memory of Claire Rayner, nurse, journalist and agony aunt.

20. Some feminists/sociologists (Knights and Morgan 1990, Shaw 1990) take issue with the use of the word 'strategy' because of its male, military connotations. Its use may presuppose that individuals have clear goals and objectives in mind when they decide how they will behave.

Although this is not always the case individuals are not passive victims shaped inevitably by circumstances and people, but have the capacity to take control over their lives. In a hierarchically structured environment such as nursing, the use of the word strategy seems particularly appropriate to describe ways in which nurses control and make choices about their social relations.

2 Putting their toe in the water: selecting, testing and expecting nurses to care

1. See Beardshaw and Robinson (1990), Section1, pp.8–12, for an analysis of the nursing work-force at the time of the first study.
2. See Note 1, Chapter 1.
3. The questionnaire was organized into five main sections, each of which covered one dimension and six to ten items or indicators of the ward learning environment. The students were asked to rate each item on a five point scale from 'strongly agree' through to 'strongly disagree'. See Companion website, Methodological Appendices I and II Ward learning Environment Questionnaire.
4. 'City' Hospital and school of nursing is a pseudonym, as are all other such proper names used in the study.
5. See Cole (1987) and Platzer (1988) for a discussion of racial and sexual discrimination in nursing recruitment and retention. See also *BMJ* editorial on black nurses, September (1988) and Hicks (1982) study of racism in nursing.
6. The Higher Education Statistics Agency (HESA) data suggested that on registration 44% of students obtained a degree and 56% obtained a diploma (HESA 2004/05). Eighty-three per cent of the questionnaire respondents were studying for a diploma and 17% for a degree.
7. During the 1960's, a minimum of two Ordinary Levels certificates of general education (GCE) were required for those undertaking training for the register. The teaching hospitals, however, had a tradition of demanding higher qualifications ranging from five 'O levels' to two Advanced Level certificates in some institutions
8. National statistics obtained in 2006 from 83 institutions, by the Nursing Standard Magazine under the Freedom of Information Act, revealed that the average attrition rate was around 26% but could vary from as low as 6% but could rise to as high as 56%. In 2008 London and the south east were reputed to have particularly high attrition rates (BBC News 2008, http://news.bbc.co.uk/1/hi/health/7337259.stm). An update at the beginning of 2010 revealed that the figures had risen to 28% in England, 11% for Northern Ireland, 20% for Wales and rising to 30% in Scotland. Measures to tackle the high drop-out rates such as 'a more sophisticated and thorough approach to selection' and 'greater financial support' were popular recommendations (www.staffnurse.com/nursing-news-articles/highest-ever-nursing-drop-out-rates-3945.html). What these recommendations suggest is that many current candidates may see nursing primarily as a paid job rather than a subject for academic study. Websites last accessed: 29 March 2011.
9. Training Body and inspectorate: The General Nursing Council of England and Wales was founded in 1919 to administer nurse training, professional practice and ward based assessment procedures similar to those undertaken by the City nurses (GNC 1969). In 1983 the Council's functions were taken over by the United Kingdom Central Council for Nursing, Midwifery and Health Visiting and four national boards, including the English National Board. This structure was then superseded by the Nursing and Midwifery Council in April 2002.
10. By September 2004, the Department of Health figures showed about 400,000 professional nurses employed in the NHS, compared to about 71,000 identified in 2000 as working in the independent sectors (Department of Health 2004a).

11. Allan et al. 2008a, Horton and Magnusson 2008, NMC 2005a, Prime Minister's Commission 2010.

3 Nothing is really said about care: defining nursing knowledge

1. See note 15, Chapter 1, on the 'New Nursing'.
2. See note 14, Chapter 1, on the nursing process as philosophy and work method.
3. During critical incident sessions, students drew on incidents from their ward experiences in order to learn about their feelings, behaviour and attitudes. The underlying assumption of the technique was that, by exploring in detail incidents from their daily work, the students could assess the influence their attitudes had on standard of care.
4. From January 1981, all general nursing students spent an 8–12-week allocation in psychiatric nursing. Research showed that in the short-term, students gained confidence in their abilities to recognize and care for patients with mental illness. However, Collister (1983) found that only four months later, when the students had returned to general nursing, these abilities were lost. The problems of applying and reinforcing skills learnt in the psychiatric setting to the general wards arose because of the diversity of the two cultures.

    An unpublished study undertaken at the same school of nursing shortly after I completed the first study confirmed these findings. During psychiatric placements, students were able to identify various skills they had learned. Third-year students who had completed their psychiatric placement one year previously could only identify talking to patients and dealing with aggression as skills they had learnt. The students on placement identified listening skills, non-verbal communication, empathy and observational skills. They were keen to take these skills back to general nursing, while the third-year students, now back in general wards prioritized patients' physical over their psychological needs.
5. The students tended to see knowledge as facts that had to be formally taught, which were different to what they did. Eraut offers alternative approaches to conceptualizing knowledge and the teaching-learning process, which are more appropriate to the students' accounts of so-called natural skills and informal learning. Knowledge also consists of unformulated tacit rules. Eraut distinguishes between technical knowledge, which is written and codified, and practical knowledge, which is expressed only in practice and learned through 'doing'. Practical knowledge is uncodified and transmitted through tone, feel and expression (1985, p. 119), like the students' accounts of *just* learning, 'picking up', 'watching', a set of hitherto uncodified caring skills.
6. The idea of teaching nurses to care evokes a heated reaction because of a concern that by learning to manage feelings they will appear false and insincere. Hochschild (1983) is also uncomfortable about the content of the training programmes on emotional labour, to which the flight attendants were exposed. She observed that, potentially, these training programmes de-skilled the flight attendants in that their personal repertoire of feelings and reactions in encounters with passengers became circumscribed by their training programmes.

4 You learn from what's wrong with the patient: defining nursing work

1. Traditionally, student nurses' allocation has been based on medical specialties. Roper (1975) undertook a study to examine the clinical content of the areas to which students were allocated.

She observed both students and patients, and examined the nursing records in order to establish the learning content available on each ward. Roper discovered that sometimes patients' diagnostic labels were different from the designated specialty of the ward. It also appeared that any patient, irrespective of diagnosis, provided nurses with teaching and learning. Roper concluded that it was difficult to predict learning experience on the basis of medical specialty. She decided therefore to develop a patient profile instrument based on Henderson's (1960) living activities. She showed how her instrument could be used as an alternative to medical diagnosis to define student learning and to plan allocation related to patient dependency and nursing needs.

2. In the first study, students undertook specialist modules in their second year and these were designed to give them a variety of experiences other than general medical and surgical nursing. These modules included placements on a number of specialist wards such as obstetrics, paediatrics, care of the elderly and psychiatry and represented a period away from what some students saw as mainstream nursing, while others enjoyed the exposure to different types of patients and work priorities.

    In the 2000s, the NMC specified that 'theoretical and practical instruction...must include nursing in relation to general and specialist medicine; general and specialist surgery; child care and paediatrics; maternity care; mental health and psychiatry; care of the old and geriatrics and home nursing'. The curriculum tends to be organized in such a way that students may be exposed to any of these specialties throughout their three years rather than just in their second year although there was a general observation by both qualified staff and students that if the students were placed with district nurses visiting patients in their home they often found returning to the acute wards, 'a culture shock' which they regarded in a similar way to how their predecessors had perceived 'mainstream nursing'.

3. The students who took part in the 2007 survey were studying adult nursing (77%) mental health (14%) and children's nursing (9%). These percentages were largely consistent with the national profile.

4. Fretwell (1982) found a similar pecking order in the students' ratings of their learning environment according to medical specialties.

5. Experimental forms of nurse training have been in operation since the 1950s, including a number of university and polytechnic programmes (MacGuire 1980). I was a student on one of these undergraduate programmes in the late 1960s. The content and structure of the course promoted a holistic and integrated approach to health care. Even so, the practice I encountered on the wards was medically driven. Despite the 'New Nursing' (see note 15, Chapter 1) the situation showed little change when in the mid-1980s I supervised undergraduate nursing students in the clinical areas.

6. These are similar findings to those of Melia (1982), Fretwell (1982) and Alexander (1983) who found that students categorized 'basic nursing' as low status work with little learning value. 'Technical nursing' had high prestige and learning value. Melia found that students classified 'patients' who required predominantly 'social' care as 'not really nursing'.

7. The Maidstone and Tunbridge Wells enquiry into the Colstridium Difficile outbreak reported in 2007 on the effects of rapid patient turnover as a factor in hospital acquired infection.

8. Statutory training days required all staff to undertake moving and handling and health and safety courses on an annual basis.

9. Two studies show how important role modelling and socialization processes are in student learning. Ousey (2006) investigated how students learned nursing and showed how students described becoming a *real* nurse through learning fundamental skills from observing and working with health care assistants. For the observing students, trained nurses were assessors, planners and evaluators and managers of care. Students could not identify who they should learn from and what they should learn; this led to a theory/practice gap and an idealization of

theory by students. Trained nurses acknowledged the theory–practice gap and said they did not practice in the way students were taught in the university. Bradshaw argues nursing has developed a culture of managing rather than delivering basic care (Bradshaw 2000). Ousey also raises issues related to what student nurses see as nursing work and whether it includes delivering as well as managing care?

10. Strauss and colleagues (1982) describe how medical legitimization shapes the nature of the work that nurses and others do in the 'technologized hospital'. Different tasks are distributed among workers, and involve two types of relationships: one is instrumental for carrying out physical and technical tasks with the patient; the other is expressive, concerning patients' psychosocial care. Strauss and colleagues have coined the term 'sentimental work' to describe and specify the content of 'psychosocial care'.

Seven categories of sentimental work were generated from data collected during field observations and interviews. Strauss and colleagues suggest their typology is useful for specifying the 'conditions, consequences and tactics' of the much used but vague term of 'working psychologically' with patients. Nurses are more likely to undertake certain types of sentimental work. As staff were not held accountable for doing sentimental work, nor was it necessarily an ingredient of trajectory work, the work was often carried out on an *ad hoc* basis. Unless it was documented or verbally reported, sentimental work remained invisible.

11. In Chapter 6 I report further on recent student responses to similar questionnaire items related to stress and anxiety and caring for dying and deceased patients and their relatives. Their responses also describe what the students experienced as the nature of the experience itself but also the lack of support from qualified staff at this time.

12. In an extensive critique of the literature on 'good' and 'bad' patients Kelly and May (1982) also found that patients with certain illnesses, diseases and symptoms were more or less popular with doctors and nurses. Their popularity also depended on their age, gender, race and class characteristics. The most popular patients were young and suffering from curable illnesses which responded to specific medical and nursing skills. See also Stockwell, 1972.

Kelly and May found that the notion of a 'caring' nurse was dependent on the notion of an 'appreciative' patient, one who confirmed the role of the nurse. Patients who denied that legitimization were seen as 'bad patients'.

In relation to my first study, this observation is important, since it suggests that students found it easier to undertake emotional labour, i.e. appear more caring towards patients whom they liked. The story of Mr Bear illustrates this point very clearly. Emotional labour costs less when the patient is appreciative.

13. Teaching on race, ethnicity and culture was relatively weak at the City Hospital during the period of the study. This improved slightly following the introduction of an equal opportunities policy. Despite the more people-centred approach of Project 2000, there is still some criticism of nurse education in general for its lack of attention to race and ethnicity within the curriculum. See Mohammed (1986).

14. General conventions used in the UK use the term 'ethnic minority group' to refer to minority populations of non-White status – for example, South Asian including populations originating from India, Pakistan, Bangladesh and Sri Lanka; East Asian, including populations originating from China, Japan and Malaysia; African, in particular sub-Saharan Africa, African American and African Caribbean (also described as 'Black'); 'White', the term usually used to describe populations originating from countries of the European community, including the UK and Ireland.

15. Issues of multiculturalism in the contemporary nursing workforce are discussed in Allan, H. T. and Smith, P. A. (2009), 'Turning a Blind Eye to Overseas Nurses' Needs: "Troublesome" Individuals and "Troubled" Institutions Or the Cultural Context of Communication: Overseas Nurses' Experience of Being "Different" in the NHS', in Bryan K (ed.) *Communication in Healthcare*, ICS, London.

16. Lofmark & Wikblad (2001) found that students appreciated reflective sessions because they helped them process and make sense of their emotional learning, what Eraut (2008) calls their 'immersive experiences'.

5 The ward sister and the infrastructure of emotion work: making it visible on the ward – from ward sister to ward manager and the role of the mentor

1. The majority of the long stay institutions described during the sixties, seventies and eighties have since been dismantled and a variety of community-based initiatives set up to take their place.
2. See Agenda for Change and KSF frameworks.
3. The RCN investigation of the role of the ward sister/charge nurse (2009) found that many staff nurses saw the role as less attractive compared with the status and pay offered by becoming a specialist nurse.
4. The 'hub' and 'spokes' practice experience referred to the way in which placements were organized to give students opportunities to see how the multidisciplinary team worked across disciplines and beyond.

6 Death and dying in hospital: the ultimate emotional labour

1. I was aware of and had read a number of studies about dying before I first wrote this chapter in 1990. These studies included Glaser and Strauss's (1965, 1970) work: *Awareness of Dying* and *Anguish: A Case History of a Dying Trajectory*, and David Field's *Nursing, the Dying* (1989). I also talked to Nicky James and read her work on hospice care. All are fine works and undoubtedly heightened my sensitivity and drew my attention to particular aspects of death and dying in hospital. For example, Glaser and Strauss (1965, 1970) address three key issues which are apparent in the structure of my chapter: (1) how death and dying are defined in hospital and the uncertainty surrounding if, when and how it will occur; (2) how the patient's dying trajectory is systematized and managed by hospital personnel given the unpredictability of death (patients can alternate between 'certain to die on time' and 'lingering reprieve'); and (3) accountable and non-accountable aspects of terminal care. Nurses were held accountable for physical care, observation of vital signs and pain relief, which often increased as death approached. No member of staff was held accountable for psychosocial aspects of care, with the result that the 'demanding' patient of their case study became more isolated as death approached.
2. Glaser and Strauss's notion of sentimental (see note 10, Chapter 4) order, for example, is very important in terms of how the feeling rules of a ward are shaped by the medical as well as the nursing agenda. The sentimental order is associated with the number of deaths expected to take place on a ward. Glaser and Strauss found that involvement with patients was encouraged on those wards with low expectation of death. Because death was an infrequent event and because nurses became involved with patients, they were extremely upset when any of them died. On wards which cared for cancer patients of intensive therapy units, where the death rate was high, the sentimental order of the ward discouraged patient involvement. Nurses learnt to maintain their composure during the dying process and transfer their involvement to the patients' relatives.

Times have changed since Glaser and Strauss first reported their findings (1965). There is now a greater recognition, by society in general and health carers in particular, that the psychological impact of death and dying must be acknowledged, especially in oncology wards and hospices, but not necessarily on general wards.

3. This is an example of surface acting. The student said she felt sad because she thought that was how she should feel.

4. Was the student deep acting, in that, because she knew the patient, she could really feel her suffering and knew how to comfort her?

5. Benner and Wrubel believe that one way of overcoming the problem described by the patient i.e. to prevent getting involved', is to see people in a context (1989, p. 48).

  The authors draw on Heideggerian philosophy and a phenomenological perspective to view the person as neither subject nor object. The person (the nurse), through concern (an essential part of human existence), is involved in the other (the patient). This involvement means that the world is understood in the light of the concern. The person is defined by her concerns which involves her in the other. In the philosophical sense the need to prevent involvement is not an issue. But in the empirical reality, conditions may be such that the nurse is prevented from becoming involved.

6. Holman C. (2008) *International Journal of Older People Nursing* 3, 278–281, 'Living Bereavement: An Exploration of Healthcare Workers' Responses to Loss and Grief in an NHS Continuing Care Ward for Older People'.

  This article reports on research rooted in a work-based education project, and the theme of loss was chosen by the participating care staff who felt it was central to their work with dependent older people. They coined the phrase 'living bereavement', meaning the complex responses and grief reactions of those experiencing and bearing witness to the multiple losses endured in continuing care environments. The aim of the research was to identify the emotional demand of living bereavement and to explore and develop care staff's capacity to work with it. The key message from the findings was explained as an intense emotional demand in care work related to loss and grief in continuing care environments. It was suggested that the emotional aspects of care work were glossed over or ignored, which affected the way care was delivered. This may have been because the feelings were disturbing or painful to deal with. It is important to support staff working with difficult feelings so that emotional aspects of their work can be acknowledged and thought about.

7. Marie Curie Palliative Care Institute, Liverpool Care Pathway, 2007.

8. In England, of the 500,000 people who die each year, 58% die in hospital, 18% in their own homes, 17% in residential homes, 4% in hospices and 3% elsewhere (2007 figures).

9. Chapter 1 features the second year student in the original study who expressed surprise that none of the trained staff actually asked her whether she was managing to cope as a young inexperienced nurse with caring for a dying child who 'took to me' and her family.

10. In the first study a student, only weeks into her training, soon realized that the running of a hospital was in opposition to the people-centred ethos of the nursing process and hence a more nurturing approach to patient care current at the time. She said: 'I mean hospitals aren't run for the individual patient, they're run for everybody, aren't they? It would be nice if they could be geared to each person but they can't really, can they?'

7 The caring trajectory: caring styles and capacity over time

1. In November 2010 the NHS Ombudsman's report revealed that the care of elderly surgical patients was 'failing to treat them with care and respect' and that a particular area of concern was the lack of effective pain control.

The NHS Ombudsman's Report, November 2010, www.bbc.co.uk/news/ health-12464831, last accessed: 3 April 2011.
2. See note 5, Chapter 3.
3. The Mid-Staffordshire Inquiry, which first reported in 2009 followed by a public inquiry in 2010, was met by media coverage asking whether student nurses and their tutors could have done more to expose the incidents of gross negligence and poor patient care.
4. See the discussion of how emotional labour and emotional intelligence relate to each other (Huy 1999) and elaborated by Freshwater and Stickley (2004) in terms of the educational curriculum.
5. See Chapter 1 for a discussion of how nurses manage anxiety (Menzies 1960).
6. This finding concurred with Brown (1973), who, from a study of long-stay hospital wards, concluded that only by providing strong social support could the deeply felt humanitarian views present in most hospital workers become effective and prevent the development or acceptance of beliefs that dehumanized patients.

8 Conclusions

1. Nursing Narratives Conference, University of Edinburgh, 11 March 2010, http://www.ed.ac. uk/schools-departments/health/nursing-studies/research/seminars, last accessed: 3 March 2011.
2. In Agenda for Change, the other job evaluation factors emphasized competences for the job and governance issues, in particular responsibility and accountability: 2. Knowledge, training and experience; 3. Analytical skills; 4.Planning & organizational skills; 5. Physical skills; 6. Responsibility – patient/client care; 7. Responsibility – policy & service; 8. Responsibility – financial & physical 9. Responsibility – HR; 10. Responsibility – Information resources; 11. Responsibility – research; 12. Freedom to act; 13. Physical effort; 14. Mental effort; 16. Working conditions.
3. In 2008 the participation of nurse and midwife academics in the Research Assessment Exercise was very successful as a result of investment in research infrastructure, funding and postgraduate education (http://www.guardian.co.uk/education/2008/dec/18/nursing-rae-research/print, last accessed: 4 February 2011).

References

Abel-Smith, B. (1960) *A History of the Nursing Profession* (London: Heinemann).

Akerjordet, K. and Severinsson, E. (2004) 'Emotional Intelligence in Mental Health Nurses Talking about Practice', *International Journal Mental Health Nursing*, 13, 3, 164–70.

Alexander, M. F. (1983) *Learning to Nurse* (Edinburgh: Churchill Livingstone).

Alexander, Z. and Dewjee, A. (1984) *Wonderful Adventures of Mrs Seacole in Many Lands* (London: Falling Wall Press).

Allan, H. (2007) 'The Rhetoric of Caring and the Recruitment of Overseas Nurses: The Social Production of a Care Gap', *Journal of Clinical Nursing*, 16, 12, 2221–8.

Allan, H. and Larsen, A. J. (2003) *'We Need Respect': Experiences of Internationally Recruited Nurses in the UK*, London RCN (publication code 002 061), http://www.rcn.org.uk/__data/assets/pdf_file/0008/78587/002061.pdf, last accessed: 28 February 2011.

Allan, H, Smith, P, O'Driscoll, M. and Lorentzon, M (2008a) *Leadership for Learning: A Review of the Literature and a Case Study into Whether Changes in Nurse Education and Health Care Organisation Have Influenced the Ways in Which Student Nurses Learn in the New NHS*, End of Project Report. (London: General Nursing Council Trust for England and Wales and Guildford: Centre for Research in Nursing and Midwifery Education, University of Surrey).

Allan H. T., Smith P. A., Lorentzon, M. (2008b) 'Leadership for Learning: A Literature Study of Leadership for Learning in Clinical Practice', *Journal of Nursing Management* 16: 545–55.

Allan H. T., Cowie, H. and Smith, P. (2009) 'Overseas Nurses' Experiences of Discrimination: A Case of Racist Bullying?' *Journal of Nursing Management*, 17, 7, 898–906.

Archer, M. (2000) *Being Human: The Problem of Agency* (Cambridge: Cambridge University Press).

Armstrong, D. (1983) 'The Fabrication of Nurse-Patient Relationships', *Social Science and Medicine*, 14B, 3–13.

Ars Vivendi (2009) *Symposium Report: Logic and Ethics of Care: Nursing Care, Emotion and Labour*, Global Centre of Excellence (COE) Programme Ars Vivendi. (Ritsumeikan University, Kyoto: Research Centre for Ars Vivendi, Ritsumeikan University).

Bate, P. and Robert, G. (2007) 'Toward More User Centric OD: Lessons from the Field of Experience Based Design and a Case Study', *Journal of Applied Behavioural Science*, 43, 41–66.

Batty, D. (2010) 'Healthy concerns, Public', *Guardian*, February 8th citing NHS Health and Well Being: the Boorman Review (2009) http://www.guardianpublic.co.uk/nhs-staff-sickness-roundtable-benenden-ealtchare, last accessed: 4th February 2011.

Baxter, C. (1988) *The Black Nurse: An Endangered Species* (Cambridge: National Extension College for Race and Health)

Beardshaw, V. and Robinson, R. (1990) *New For Old? Prospects for Nursing in the 1990s* (London: King's Fund Institute).

Bell, C. and Roberts, H. (eds) (1984) *Social Researching – Politics, Problems, Practice* (London: Routledge and Kegan Paul).

Bellaby, P. and Oribabor, P. (1980) 'The History of the Present – Contradiction and Struggle in Nursing', in Davies, C. (ed.) *Rewriting Nursing History*, pp. 147–173 (London: Croom Helm).

Bellack J (1999) 'Emotional Intelligence: A Missing Ingredient?' *Journal of Nursing Education* 38, 1, 3–4.

Benner, P. (1984) *From Novice to Expert – Excellence and Power in Clinical Nursing Practice* (Menlo Park, CA: Addison-Wesley).

Benner, P. and Wrubel, R. (1989) *The Primacy of Caring: Stress and Coping in Health and Illness* (Menlo Park, CA: Addison-Wesley).

Benton, D. (2004) 'Sharing best practice across the Atlantic', *Nursing Times* 100, 4, 26–7.

Bolton, S. C. (2000) 'Who Cares? Offering Emotion Work as a "Gift in the Nursing Labour Process"', *Journal of Advanced Nursing*, 32, 580–6.

Bolton, S. C. (2001) 'Changing Faces: Nurses as Emotional Jugglers'. *Sociology of Health and Illness*, 23, 85–100.

Bolton, S. and Boyd, C. (2003) 'Trolley Dolly Or Skilled Emotion Manager? Moving on from Hochschild's Managed Heart', *Work, Employment and Society* 17, 2, 289–308.

Bone, D. (2009) 'Epidurals Not Emotions: the Care Deficit in US Maternity Care'. In Hunter B and Deery R (eds) *Emotions in Midwifery and Reproduction* (Basingstoke: Palgrave Macmillan), 56–70.

Bostridge, M. (2008) *Florence Nightingale: The Woman and her Legend* (London: Viking).

Bracken, E. and Davis, J. (1989) 'The Implication of Mentorship in Nursing Career Development', *Senior Nurse*, 9, 5, 15–16.

Bradshaw, A. (2000) 'Competence and British Nursing: a View from History', *Journal of Clinical Nursing*, 9, 3, 321–9.

Bray, L. and Nettleton, P. (2007) 'Assessor Or Mentor? Role Confusion in Professional Education', *Nurse Education Today*, 27, 848–55.

Brindle, D. (1990) 'A Happy Ward with No Nurses', *Guardian*, 14 September.

Brindle, D. (2010) 'Whistle-Blowing Cloud Over Students at Scandal Hospital', *Guardian*, 2 November.

British Medical Journal (1988) 'Black Nurses', *British Medical Journal*, 297, 639.

Brooks L. (2011) 'The Taming of Jane Goody', *Guardian*, 11 February.

Brown, G. W. (1973) 'The Mental Hospital as An Institution', *Social Science and Medicine*, 7, 407–24.

Bulmer, M. (1983) 'Concepts in the Analysis of Qualitative Data', in Bulmer, M. (ed.) *Sociological Research Methods: An Introduction*, 2nd edn (London: Macmillan).

Carpenter, M. (1977) 'The New Managerialism and Professionalism in Nursing', in Stacey, M., Reid, M., Heath, C, and Dingwall, R, (eds) *Health and the Division of Labour*, pp. 165–193 (London: Croom Helm).

Carpenter, M. (1978) 'Managerialism and the Division of Labour in Nursing', in Dingwall, R. and McKintosh, J. (eds) *Readings in the Sociology of Nursing*, pp. 87–103 (Edinburgh: Churchill Livingstone).

Carvel, J. (2008) 'Nurses to Be Rated on How Compassionate and Smiley They Are', *Guardian*, 18 June.

Chambers, C. and Ryder, E. (2009) *Compassion and Caring in Nursing* (Oxford: Radcliffe Publishing)

Choy, C.C. (2003) *Empire of Care: Nursing and Migration in Filipino American History* (Durham: Duke University Press)

Clamp, C. (1980) 'Learning through Incidents', *Nursing Times*, 76, 40, 1755–8.

Clouder, L. (2005) 'Caring as a Threshold Concept: Transforming Students in Higher Education into Health(Care) Professionals', *Teaching in Higher Education*, 10, 4, 505–17.

Cole, A. (1987) 'Racism, Limited Access', *Nursing Times and Nursing Mirror*, 83, 24, 29–30.

Collins, H. M. (1974) 'The TEA Set: Tacit Knowledge and Scientific Networks', *Science Studies*, 4, 165–86.

Collins, H. M. (1984) 'Researching Spoonbending: Concepts and Practice of Participatory Fieldwork', in Bell, C. and Roberts, H. (eds) *Social Researching – Politics, Problems, Practice*, pp. 54–69 (London: Routledge and Kegan Paul).

Collister, B. (1983) 'The Value of Psychiatric Experience in General Nurse Training', *Nursing Times*, Occasional Papers, 79, 29, 66–9.

Cornwell, J. and Goodrich, J. (2009) 'Exploring How to Ensure Compassionate Care in Hospital to Improve Patient Experience', *Nursing Times*, 105, 15, 14–16.

Coser, R. L. (1962) *Life on the Ward* (East Lansing, MI: Michigan State University Press).

Davies, C. (1976) 'Experience of Dependency and Control in Work: the Case of Nurses', *Journal of Advanced Nursing*, 1, 273–82.

Davies, C. and Rosser, J. (1986) 'Gendered Jobs in the Health Service: a Problem for Labour Process Analysis', in Knight, D. and Wilmott, H. (eds.) *Gender and the Labour Process*, pp. 94–116 (Aldershot: Gower).

Davies, K. (1990) *Women, Time and the Weavings of the Strands of Everyday Life* (Aldershot: Avebury).

de la Cuesta, C. (1983) 'The Nursing Process: From Development to Implementation', *Journal of Advanced Nursing*, 8, 365–71.

Denzin, N. (1970) 'Strategies of Multiple Triangulation', in *The Research Act in Sociology* (London: Butterworth).

Department of Health (1990) *Nurse Recruitment* (London: HMSO).

Department of Health (1999) *Making a Difference* (London: Department of Health).

Department of Health (2000) *The NHS Plan: A Plan for Investment, a Plan for Reform*, (London: Department of Health).

Department of Health (2001) *The Essence of Care: Patient-Focused Benchmarking for Health Care Practitioners* (London: Department of Health).

Department of Health (2003a) *Delivering the HR in the NHS Plan*. (London: Department of Health).

Department of Health (2003b) *New Ways of Working* (London: NHS Modernization Agency, Department of Health).

Department of Health (2004a) *Agenda for Change: Final Agreement* (London: Department of Health).

Department of Health (2004b) *The NHS Knowledge and Skills Framework and the Development Review Process: Final Draft* (London: Department of Health).

Department of Health (2004c) *National Standards, Local Action: Health and Social Care Standards and Planning Framework 2005/06–2007/08* (London: Department of Health).

Department of Health (2006) *Modernising Nursing Careers – Setting the Direction*. (London: Department of Health).

Department of Health (2007) *Towards a Framework for Post Registration Nursing Careers: Consultation Document*. (London: Department of Health).

Department of Health (2008) *High Quality Care for All* (London: The Stationery Office).

Department of Health (2010a) *Equity and Excellence: Liberating the NHS*. (London: Department of Health).

Department of Health (2010b) *Preceptorship Framework for Newly Registered Nurses, Midwives and Allied Health Professionals* (London: Department of Health).

Department of Health and Social Security (1972) *Report of the Committee on Nursing* (Chair: A. Briggs) (London: HMSO).

Dewar, B. J. and Macleod-Clark, J. (1992) 'The Role of the Paid Non-Professional Nursing Helper: A Review of the Literature', *Journal of Advanced Nursing*, 17, 1, 113–20.

Dewar, B., Mackay, R., Smith, S., Pullin, S. and Tocher, R. (2010) 'Use of Emotional Touch Points as a Method of Tapping into the Experiences of Receiving Compassionate Care in a Hospital Setting', *Journal of Research in Nursing*, 15, 29–41 (online version, http://jrn.sagepub.com/cgi/content/abstract/15/1/29)

Einarsen, S. (2004) 'Victimisation from Bullying at Work: We Need to Understand the Process', *Occupational Health Psychologist*, 11, 11, 4–5.

English National Board (1987) *Circular* 1987/28/MAT.

Eraut, M. (1985) 'Knowledge Creation and Knowledge Use in Professional Contexts' *Studies in Higher Education*, 10, 2, 117–33.

Eraut, M. Steadman, S. Maillardet, F. and Miller, C. (2007) *Early Career Learning at Work: Insights into Professional Development during the First Job*. Economic and Social Research Council Teaching and Learning Research Programme, Teaching and Learning Research Briefing, March, no. 25, www.tlrp.org/pub/research.html, last accessed: 4 February 2011.

Evans, K., Guile, D. and Harris, J. (2009) *Putting Knowledge to Work: Integrating Work-Based and Subject-Based Knowledge in Intermediate Level Qualifications and Workforce Upskilling*. (London: The Work-based learning for education environments [WLE] Centre, Institute of Education).

Evans, K., Guile, J. and Allan, H. (2010) 'Putting Knowledge to Work: A New Approach', *Nurse Education Today*, 30, 3, 245–51.

Evers, H. (1981a) 'Tender Loving Care? Patients and Nurses in Geriatric Wards', in Copp, L. A. (ed.) *Care of the Ageing* (Edinburgh: Churchill Livingstone).

Evers, H. (1981b) 'Care Or Custody? The Experiences of Women Patients in Long-Stay Geriatric Wards', in Williams, G. and Hutter, B. (eds) *Controlling Women – the Normal and the Deviant* (London: Croom Helm).

Evers, H. K. (1984) *Patients' Experiences and Social Relations in Geriatric Wards* (Ph.D. thesis: University of Warwick).

Field, D. (1989) *Nursing the Dying* (London: Tavistock/Routledge).

Flax, J. (1987) 'Postmodernism and Gender Relations in Feminist Theory', *Signs: Journal of Women in Culture and Society*, 12, 4, 621–43.

Fox, R. (1959) *Experiment Perilous* (Glencoe, IL: Free Press of Glencoe).

Francis, R. (2010a) *Independent Inquiry into Care Provided by Mid Staffordshire NHS Foundation Trust January 2005– March 2009 Volumes I and II, chaired by Robert Francis QC* (London: The Stationery Office).

Francis, R. (2010b) Speech at the launch of the *Final Report of The Independent Inquiry Into Care Provided by Mid Staffordshire NHS Foundation Trust*, 02 March 2010, http://www.midstaffsinquiry.com/news.php, accessed 11 September 2011.

Freidson, E. (1970) *The Profession of Medicine: A Study of the Sociology of Applied Knowledge* (New York: Dodd, Mead and Co.).

Freshwater, D. and Stickley, T. (2004) 'The Heart of the Art: Emotional Intelligence in Nurse Education' *Nursing Inquiry*, 11, 91–8.

Fretwell, J. E. (1982) *Ward Teaching and Learning: Sister and the Learning Environment* (London: Royal College of Nursing).

Fretwell, J. E. (1985) *Freedom to Change* (London: Royal College of Nursing).

General Nursing Council Communication 69/4/3 Paper C (1969) *Changes Proposed in the Final State Examination* (London: General Nursing Council).

General Nursing Council for England and Wales (1977) *Training Syllabus. Register of Nurses: General Nursing* (London: General Nursing Council for England and Wales).

Gilligan, C. (1982) *In a Different Voice* (Cambridge, MA: Harvard University Press).

Glaser, B. G. and Strauss, A. L. (1965) *Awareness of Dying* (Chicago: Aldine).

Glaser, B. and Strauss, A. (1967) *The Discovery of Grounded Theory* (London: Weidenfeld & Nicolson).

Goddard, H. A. (1953) *The Work of Nurses in Hospital Wards: Report of a Job Analysis* (Oxford: Nuffield Provincial Hospitals Trust).

Goffman, E. (1968) *Asylums* (Harmondsworth: Penguin).

Gold, R. L. (1969) 'Roles in Sociological Field Observations', in McCall, G. J. and Simmons, J. L. (eds) *Issues in Participant Observation: a Text and Reader* (Reading, MA: Addison-Wesley).

Goleman, D. P. (1995) *Emotional Intelligence: Why It Can Matter More Than IQ for Character, Health and Lifelong Achievement* (New York: Bantam Books).

Gordon, S. (1988) 'Giving Nurses Time to Care', *Washington Post*, 6 September.

Graham, H. (1983) 'Caring: a Labour of Love', in Finch, J. and Groves, D. (eds) *A Labour of Love: Women, Work and Caring* (London: Routledge and Kegan Paul).

Croun, C. (2010) 'Memorial to Crimea's Black Nurse in Danger', *Independent*, 25 January.

Hayward, J. (1975) *Information: A Prescription Against Pain* (London. Royal College of Nursing).

Health Care Commission (2007) *Investigation into Outbreaks of Clostridium difficile at Maidstone and Tunbridge Wells NHS Trust.* (London: HCC).

Health Care Commission (2008) *National Survey of NHS Staff*, Commission for Health Care Audit and Inspection, http://www.nhsstaffsurveys.com last accessed 28 June 2009.

Henderson, V. (1960) *Basic Principles of Nursing Care* (Geneva: International Council of Nurses).

Hicks, C. (1982) 'Racism in Nursing', *Nursing Times*, 78, 18, 743–8.

Higher Education Statistics Agency (HESA) (2004/5) http://www.hesa.ac.uk/dox/dataTables/studentsAndQualifiers/download/quals0405.xls, last accessed: 30 January 2011.

Hochschild, A. R. (1983) *The Managed Heart: Commercialisation of Human Feeling* (Berkeley: University of California Press).

Hochschild, A. (1989) *The Second Shift: Working Parents and the Revolution at Home* (New York: Viking/Penguin).

Hochschild A. R. (2003) *The Commercialisation of Intimate Life* (Berkeley: University of California Press).

Hockey, J. (1990) *Experience of Death: An Anthropological Account.* (Edinburgh: Edinburgh University Press).

Holman, C. (2008) 'Living Bereavement: An Exploration of Healthcare Workers' Responses to Loss and Grief in An NHS Continuing Care Ward for Older People', *International Journal of Older People Nursing*, 3, 278–81.

Horton, K. and Magnusson, C. (2008) *A Review of Student Exit Interview Processes. Final Report* (Guildford: Centre for Research in Nursing and Midwifery Education (CRNME), University of Surrey).

Huy, Q.N. (1999) 'Emotional Capability, Emotional Intelligence and Radical Change', *Academy of Management Review*, 24, 325–46.

James, N. (1984) 'A postscript to nursing', in Bell, C. and Roberts, H. (eds) *Social Researching – Politics, Problems, Practice* (London: Routledge and Kegan Paul).

James, N. (1989) 'Emotional Labour, Skills and Work in the Social Regulation of Feeling', *Sociological Review*, 37, 1, 15–42.

James, V. (1986) *Care and Work in Nursing the Dying* (Ph.D. thesis: University of Aberdeen).

Johns, C. (1990) 'Autonomy of Primary Nurses: The Need to Both Facilitate and Limit Autonomy in Practice', *Journal of Advanced Nursing* 15, 886–94.

Johnson, M., Ormandy, P., Long, A. F, and Hulme, C. (2004) 'Nurses' and Senior Support Workers' Views of Role and Accountability', *Intensive and Critical Care Nursing*, 20, 123–32.

Jones, A. and Bamford, O. (1998) 'Nursing Development Units: Perspectives and Prospects for Research and Practice', in Smith P (ed.) (1998) *Nursing Research Setting New Agendas*, pp. 187–211 (London: Hodder Headlines Group).

Kelly, M. P. and May, D. (1982) 'Good and Bad Patients: A Review of the Literature and a Theoretical Critique', *Journal of Advanced Nursing*, 7, 2, 147–57 (see particularly p. 154).

Kendall, M. G. and Stuart, A. (1968) *The Advanced Theory of Statistics*, 3, 2nd edn, 43–6 (London: Charles Griffin and Co.).

King, R. D., Raynes, N. V. and Tizard, J. (1971) *Patterns of Residential Care: Sociological Studies in Institutions for Handicapped Children* (London: Routledge and Kegan Paul).

Kitson, A. L. (1996) 'Does Nursing Have a Future?' *British Medical Journal*, 313, 1647–51.

Knibb, W., Smith, P., Magnusson, C. and Bryan, K. (2006) *The Contribution of Assistants to Nursing. Final Report for the Royal College of Nursing* (Guildford: Healthcare Workforce Research Centre and Centre for Research in Nursing and Midwifery Education, University of Surrey).

Knights, D. and Morgan, G. (1990) 'The Concept of Strategy in Sociology: A Note of Dissent', *Sociology* 24, 3, 475–83.

Lawton, J. (2000) *The Dying Process: Patients' Experiences of Palliative Care* (London: Routledge).

Lipsett, A. (2008) 'Nursing Research Takes Its Place on the World Stage', *Guardian* 18December, http://www.guardian.co.uk/education/2008/dec/18/nursing-rae-research/print,last accessed: 5 February 2010.

Lofmark, A. and Wikblad, K. (2001) 'Facilitating and obstructing factors for development of learning in clinical practice: a student perspective', *Journal of Advanced Nursing*, 34, 1, 43–50.

Lowes, R. (2010) Largest Ever Nurses' Strike Could be Sign of Future Unrest, *Medscape Medical News*, www.medscape.com/viewarticle/723437?src=mp&mp&spon=24&uac=97043HZ, last accessed 17 June 2010.

Magnusson, C., O'Driscoll, M. and Smith, P. (2007) 'New Roles to Support Practice Learning – Can They Facilitate Expansion of Placement Capacity?' *Nurse Education Today*, 27, 643–50.

Mann, H. (1998) 'Reflections on a Border Crossing: from Ward Sister to Clinical Nurse Specialist', in Smith P (ed.) (1998) *Nursing Research Setting New Agendas*, pp. 160–86 (London: Hodder Headlines Group).

McClure, R. and Murphy C. (2007) 'Contesting the Dominance of Emotional Labour in Professional Nursing' *Journal of Health Organisation and Management*, 21, 2, 101–20.

McFarlane, J. K. (1976) 'A Charter for Caring', *Journal of Advanced Nursing*, 1, 187–96.

McFarlane, J. K. (1977) 'Developing a Theory of Nursing: the Relation of Theory to Practice, Education and Research', *Journal of Advanced Nursing*, 2, 261–70.

MacGuire, J. (1980) 'Nursing: None Is Held in Higher Esteem. Occupational Control and the Position of Women in Nursing', in Silverstone, J. and Ward, A. (eds) *Careers of Professional Women* (London: Croom Helm).

MacMillan, P. (1980) 'Major Implications', *Nursing Times*, 76, 49, 2138–9.

Melia, K. (2006) *Nursing in the New NHS: a Sociological Analysis of Learning and Working*, ESRC Grant R000271191, http://www.esrc.ac.uk/my-esrc/Grants/R000271191/read, last accessed 28 February 2011.

Melia, K. M. (1982) '"Tell It as It Is" – Qualitative Methodology and Nursing Research: Understanding the Student Nurses' World', *Journal of Advanced Nursing*, 7, 327–35.

Melia, K. M. (1984) 'Student Nurses' Construction of Occupational Socialisation', *Sociology of Health and Illness*, 6, 2,132–49.

Melia, K. M. (1987) *Learning and Working: The Occupational Socialization of Nurses* (London: Tavistock).

Menzies, I. E. P. (1960) 'A Case Study of the Functioning of Social Systems as a Defence against Anxiety. A Report on the Study of a Nursing Service of a General Hospital', *Human Relations*, 13, 95–121.

Miller, A. and Gwynne, G. (1972) *A Life Apart* (London: Tavistock).

ModernisingNursingCareers(2011)http://www.dh.gov.uk/en/Aboutus/Chiefprofessionalofficers/Chiefnursingofficer/DH_108368, last accessed 13 February 2011.

Mohammed, S. (1986) 'A Black Perspective', *Senior Nurse*, 5, 3, 5.

Moores, B. and Moult, A. (1979) 'Patterns of Nurse Activity', *Journal of Advanced Nursing*, 4, 137–49.

Newman, M. (1994) *Health as Expanding Consciousness* (Boston: Jones and Bartlett).

Norton, D. (1962) *Investigation of Geriatric Nursing Problems in Hospitals* (Edinburgh: Churchill Livingstone).

NHS Modernisation Agency (2003) *Essence of Care: Patient-focused Benchmarks for Clinical Governance.* (London: Department of Health).

Nursing and Midwifery Admissions Service (NMAS) (2007) *Statistical Report 2006* http://www.nmas.ac.uk/stats.html, last accessed 2 April 2008.

Nursing and Midwifery Council (2004a) *Project 2000 Papers: Counting the Costs: The Final Proposals* (February 1987) (London: NMC).

Nursing and Midwifery Council (2004b) *Failing to Fail, the Duffy Report: Failing Students: A Qualitative Study of Factors That Influence the Decisions Regarding Assessment of Students' Competence in Practice* (London: NMC).

Nursing and Midwifery Council (2004c) *Standards of Proficiency for pre- registration Nursing Education* (London: NMC).

Nursing and Midwifery Council (2005a) *Statistical Analysis of the Register 1 April 2004 to 31 March 2005*, Report August 2005 (London: NMC), http://www.nmc-uk.org/nmc/main/publications/Annualstatistics20042005.pdf, last accessed: 24 October 2005.

Nursing and Midwifery Council (2005b) *Mapping Paper* (London: NMC).

Nursing and Midwifery Council (2007) NMC Circular 07/2007 *The Introduction of Essential Skills Clusters for Pre-registration Nursing Programmes.* (London: NMC).

Nursing and Midwifery Council (2008a) *Standards to Support Learning and Assessment in Practice* (London: NMC).

Nursing and Midwifery Council (2008b) *The Code: Standards of Conduct, Performance and Ethics for Nurses and Midwives* (London: NMC).

Nursing and Midwifery Council (2009) *NMC Circular 04/2009 Amendment to Standards of Proficiency for Pre- Registration Nursing Education Relating to Adult Branch Programmes and Compliance with Directive 2005/36/EC on the Recognition of Professional Qualifications* (London: NMC).

Nursing and Midwifery Council (2010a) *Nurse Education: Now and in the future: The Challenges for Nursing in the 21st Century*, (London: NMC).

Nursing and Midwifery Council (2010b) *NMC Circular 07/2010 Standards for Pre-Registration Nursing Education* (London: NMC).

Nursing and Midwifery Council (2010c) *New Options for Becoming a Sign-off Mentor, NMC Circular 05/2010 Sign-off mentor criteria*, (London: NMC).

Nursing Times (2008) Nursing Champions, *NT*, 8 December, 104, 49, www.nursingtimes.net

O'Brien, M. (1989) 'Reproducing the World', in *Reproducing the World: Essays in Feminist Theory* (USA: Westview Press).

Oakley, A. (1981) 'Interviewing Women: a Contradiction in Terms', in Roberts, H. (ed.) *Doing Feminist Research* (London: Routledge and Kegan Paul).

Oakley, A. (1984) 'The Importance of Being a Nurse', *Nursing Times*, 80, 50, 24–7.

Ogier, M. (1982) *An Ideal Sister* (London: Royal College of Nursing).

Orton, H. D. (1981) *Learning Climate: A Study of the Role of the Ward Sister in Relation to Student Nurse Learning on the Ward* (London: Royal College of Nursing).

Ousey, K. (2006) *Being a Real Nurse*, Paper presented at RCN International Research Conference. (London: Royal College of Nursing).

Parse, R. R. (1997) *The Human Becoming School of Thought: A Perspective for Nurses and Other Health Professionals* (Thousand Oaks, CA: Sage).

Pearsall, M. (1970) 'Participant Observation as Role and Method in Behaviour', in Kilstead, W. J. (ed.) *Qualitative Methodology: Firsthand Involvement with the Social World* (Chicago: Markham).

Pearson, A. (ed.) (1988) *Primary Nursing: Nursing in the Burford and Oxford Nursing Development Units* (Beckenham: Croom Helm).

Pearson, A. (2009) 'Life-changing Research', *Nursing Standard*, 23, 28, 19

Pearson, P. H., Howe, A., Steven, A., Sheik, A., Ashcroft, D., Smith, P., Bradley, F., Buckle, P., Cresswell, K., Dagley, V., Lawrence, J. and Magnusson, C. (2009) *Patient Safety in health care professional educational curricula: examining the learning experience.* Report PS 030 submitted to the Patient Safety Research Programme, Department of Health, http://www.haps.bham.ac.uk/publichealth/psrp/, *last accessed: 29 January 2011.*

Peplau, H. (1992) *Interpersonal Relations in Nursing* (London: Macmillan).

Pembrey, S. E. M. (1980) *The Ward Sister – Key to Nursing* (London: Royal College of Nursing).

Platzer, H. (1988) 'Redressing the Balance', *Nursing Standard*, 2, 15, 42.

Price Waterhouse (1988) *Nurse Recruitment and Retention: Report on the factors affecting the Retention and Recruitment of Nurses, Midwives and Health Visitors in the NHS.* Commissioned by Chairmen of Regional Health Activities in England, Health Boards in Scotland and Health Authorities in Wales. (London: Price Waterhouse).

Prime Minister's Commission (2010) *Frontline Care: The Future of Nursing and Midwifery in England. Report of the Prime Minister's Commission on the Future of Nursing and Midwifery in England* (London: Central Office of Information [COI]).

Quine, L. (1999) 'Workplace Bullying in An NHS Community Trust: Staff Questionnaire Survey', *British Medical Journal*, 318, 228–32.

Quint, J. (1967) *The Nurse and the Dying Patient* (New York: Macmillan).

Revans, R. W. (1964) *Standards for Morale: Cause and Effect in Hospitals* (Oxford: Oxford University Press).

Roper, N. (1975) *Clinical Experience in Nurse Education: A Survey of the Available Nursing Experience for General Student Nurses in a School of Nursing in Scotland* (M.Phil. thesis: University of Edinburgh).

Roper, N. (1976) 'A Model for Nursing and Nursology', *Journal of Advanced Nursing*, 1, 219–27.

Ross, F., Christian, S., Bing, R., Smith, P., Allan, H., Clayton, J., Price, L., Redfern, S., Brearley, S., Manthorpe, J. and Mackintosh, M. (2009) *The Professional Experience of Governance and Incentives: Meeting the Needs of People with Complex Conditions in Primary, May 2006 – Report Submitted to the SDO Programme, Department of Health,* http://www.sdo.nihr.ac.uk/files/project/128-final-report.pdf, last accessed 29 January 2011.

Royal College of Nursing (2005) *Agenda for Change: A Guide to the New Pay, Terms and Conditions in the NHS.* (London: Royal College Nursing).

Royal College of Nursing (2009) *Breaking Down Barriers, Driving Up Standards, the Role of the Sister and Charge Nurse* (London: Royal College of Nursing).

Ruddick, S. (1989) *Maternal Thinking: Toward a Politics of Peace* (Boston: Beacon Press).

Salvage, J. (1985) *The Politics of Nursing* (London: Heinemann).

Salvage, J. (1990) 'The Theory and Practice of the "New Nursing"', *Nursing Times*, Occasional Paper, 86, 4, 42–5.

Savage, J. (2000) 'Ethnography and healthcare', *British Medical Journal*, 321,1400–2.

Scott, H. (2004) 'Are Nurses "Too Clever to Care" and "Too Posh to Wash?"' *British Journal of Nursing* 13, 10, 581.

Sharples K (2009) *Learning to Learn in Nursing Practice* (Exeter: Learning Matters).

Shaw, M. (1990) 'Debate on the Concept of Strategy. Strategy and Social Process: Military Context and Sociological Analysis', *Sociology*, 24, 3, 465–73.

Sheehan, J. (1983) 'Educating for Teaching Nursing', in Davis, B. D. (ed.) *Research into Nurse Education* (London: Croom Helm).

Smith, P. (1987) 'The Relationship between Quality of Nursing Care and the Ward as a Learning Environment: Developing a Methodology', *Journal of Advanced Nursing*, 12, 413–20.

Smith, P. (1992) *The Emotional Labour of Nursing: How Nurses Care* (Basingstoke: Palgrave Macmillan).

Smith, P. (2008) 'Compassion and Smiles: What's the Evidence?' *Journal of Research in Nursing*, 13, 5, 367–70.

Smith, P. (2010) 'The Emotional Labour of Nursing: The Current Situation and Hereafter', *Japanese Red Cross Bulletin of Nursing*, 24, 160–70.

Smith, P. and Cowie, H. (2010) 'Perspectives on Emotional Labour and Bullying: Reviewing the Role of Emotions in Nursing and Healthcare' *International Journal of Work, Organisation and Emotion*, 3, 3, 227–236.

Smith, P. and Gray, B. (2001a) 'Emotional Labour of Nursing Revisited: Caring and Learning 2000', *Nurse Education in Practice*, 1, 42–9.

Smith, P. and Gray, B. (2001b) 'Reassessing the Concept of Emotional Labour in Student Nurse Education: Role of Link Lecturers and Mentors in a Time of Change', *Nurse Education Today*, 21 230–7.

Smith, P. and Mackintosh, M. (2007) 'Profession Market and Class: Nurse Migration and the Re-Making of Division and Disadvantage', *Journal of Clinical Nursing*, 16, 12, 2213–20.

Smith, P. Masterson, A. and Lask, S. (1995) 'Health and the Curriculum: An Illuminative Evaluation – Part II – Findings and Recommendations', *Nurse Education Today*, 15, 317–22.

Smith, P., Pearson, P.H. and Ross, F. (2009) 'Emotions at Work: What Is the Link to Patient and Staff Safety? Implications for Nurse Managers in the NHS', *Journal of Nursing Management* 17, 230–237.

Smith, P. A. (1988) *Quality of Nursing and the Ward as a Learning Environment for Student Nurses* (Unpublished PhD thesis, London: King's College, University of London).

Smith, P. A., Allan, H. T., Henry, L. W., Larsen. J. A. and Mackintosh, M. M. (2006) *Valuing and Recognizing the Talents of a Diverse Healthcare Workforce* (Guildford: The Centre for Research in Nursing and Midwifery Education, University of Surrey, Milton Keynes: The Open University and London: the Royal College of Nursing), http://www.rcn.org.uk/—data/assets/pdf_file/0008/78713/003078.pdf, last accessed 28 February 2011.

Sontag, S. (1983) *Illness as Metaphor* (Harmondsworth: Penguin).

Stacey, M. (1981) 'The Division of Labour Revisited Or Overcoming the Two Adams', in Abrams, P., Deem, R., Finch, J. and Rock, P. (eds) *Practice and Progress: British Sociology 1950–1980* (London: Allen and Unwin).

Stanley, L. and Wise, S. (1983) *Breaking Out: Feminist Consciousness and Feminist Research* (London: Routledge and Kegan Paul).

Stockwell, F. (1972) *The Unpopular Patient* (London: Royal College of Nursing).

Strauss, A., Fagerhaugh, S., Suczek, B. and Wiener, C. (1982) 'Sentimental Work in the Technologized Hospital', *Sociology of Health and Illness*, 4, 3, 254–78.

Strauss, A. L. and Glaser, B. G. (1970) *Anguish: A Case History of a Dying Trajectory* (London: Martin Robinson).

Sudnow, D. (1967) *Passing on: The Social Organisation of Dying* (Englewood Cliffs, NJ: Prentice Hall).

Takei A (2001) *Emotion and Nursing: Meaning of Caring for People as a Profession.* (Japan: Iagaku-Shoin).

Taylor, D. (2006) *What Immortal Hand or Eye Has Framed the Fearful Symmetry?* Paper presented at 'Governed States of Mind: Thinking Psychoanalytically', St Hugh's College, Oxford, UK. 24–25March 2006.

Theodosius, C. (2006) 'Recovering Emotion from Emotion Management', *Sociology*, 40, 5, 893–910.

Theodosius, C. (2008) *Emotional Labour in Health Care: the Unmanaged Heart of Nursing* (London: Routledge).

Titmuss, R. M. (1970) *The Gift Relationship: From Human Blood to Social Policy*. (London: Allen and Unwin).

Thornley, C. (2001) *'Non-Registered Nurses in the NHS – An Update'*, (London: UNISON).

Tronto, J. C. (1987) 'Beyond Gender Difference to a Theory of Care', *Signs: Journal of Women in Culture and Society*, 12, 4, 644–63.

Ungerson, C. (1983a) 'Why Do Women Care?', in Finch, J. and Groves, D. (eds) *A Labour of Love: Women, Work and Caring* (London: Routledge and Kegan Paul).

Ungerson, C. (1983b) 'Women and Caring: Skills, Tasks and Taboos', in Gamarnikov, E., Morgan, D., Purvis, J. and Taylorson, D. (eds) *The Public and the Private* (London: Heinemann).

Ungerson, C. (1990) 'The Language of Care', in Ungerson, C. (ed.) *Gender and Caring* (London: Harvester/Wheatsheaf).

United Kingdom Central Council (1999) *Fitness for Practice: The UK Commission for Nursing and Midwifery Education*. (London: UKCC).

United Kingdom Central Council for Nursing, Midwifery and Health Visiting Educational Policy Advisory Committee (1985) *Project 2000: Facing the Future. Project Paper 6* (London: UKCC).

United Kingdom Central Council for Nursing, Midwifery and Health Visiting (1986) *Project 2000: A New Preparation for Practice* (London: UKCC).

United Kingdom Central Council for Nursing, Midwifery and Health Visiting (1990) *The Post-Registration Education and Practice Project (PREPP)* (London: UKCC).

Webb, C. (1984) 'Feminist Methodology in Nursing Research', *Journal of Advanced Nursing*, 9, 249–50.

Williams, S. (1999) 'Student Carers: Learning to Manage Emotions', *Soundings*, 11, 180–6.

Web sites

http://www.macmillan.org.uk
Macmillan Cancer Support, last accessed 28 February 2011.

http://www.mariecurie.org.uk
Marie Curie Cancer Care, last accessed 28 February 2011.

http://www.napier.ac.uk/fhlss/NMSC/compassionatecare
Leadership in Compassionate Care Programme, last accessed 28 February 2011.

http://www.whitehallpages.net
(Beasley et al. 2009) 'Nursing Set to Become All Graduate Entry by 2013', created 12 November 2009, last accessed 17 May 2010.

http://www.publicservice.co.uk
(Beasley et al 2010) Degree-Only Nursing: Are Academic Achievement and Safe, Compassionate Care Mutually Exclusive? Created 1 April 2010, last accessed 17 May 2010.

http://www.napier.ac.uk/ccnews
Compassionate Care Project Reports, last accessed 28 February 2011.

http://www.rcn.org.uk/newsevents/news/article/uk/brown_and_cameron_address_delegates_ in_historic_day_at_congress
(Brown, G. 2009) Speech to RCN Congress, last accessed 28 February 2011.

http://www.lookafterournhs.org.uk
Look after our NHS (British Medical Association), last accessed 28 February 2011.

http://www.dh.gov.uk/en/Aboutus/Chiefprofessionalofficers/Chiefnursingofficer/DH_108368
'Modernising Nursing Careers', last accessed 5 February 2011.

Index